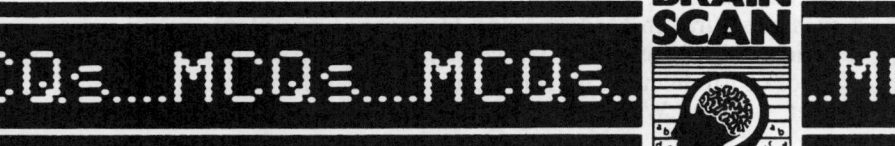

Norman Johnson · Chris Bunker

. . . more
MRCP Part 1

W0050444

Springer-Verlag
London Berlin Heidelberg New York
Paris Tokyo

Norman Johnson, MD, FRCP
Senior Lecturer in Medicine and Honorary Consultant
Physician, Middlesex and University College Hospitals
School of Medicine, The Middlesex Hospital, Mortimer
Street, London W1N 8AA, England

Chris Bunker, MA, MRCP
Registrar in Dermatology,
The Middlesex Hospital, Mortimer Street,
London W1N 8AA, England

Publisher's note: the "Brainscan" logo is reproduced by courtesy of The
Editor, *Geriatric Medicine*, Modern Medicine GB Ltd.

ISBN-13:978-3-540-19507-8   e-ISBN-13:978-1-4471-1606-6
DOI: 10.1007/978-1-4471-1606-6

British Library Cataloguing in Publication Data
Johnson, N. *1948–*
. . . More MRCP Part I
1. Medicine. Questions and answers
I. Title
610'.76
ISBN-13:978-3-540-19507-8

Filmset by Wilmaset, Birkenhead, Wirral

2128/3916–543210

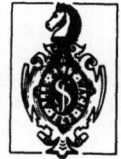

Contents

Introduction to MRCP Part I

Multiple choice questions have been a popular way of setting exams for at least 20 years. However fair or unfair they appear to be, they are destined to remain a part of the system. The main reason for their popularity is that they provide a compact method of testing the candidate's knowledge over a very wide field. This is an obvious advantage in a subject such as medicine. Multiple choice questions allow easy and unbiased marking which can be performed rapidly by computer. Computerised marking also facilitates qualitative control of questions and statistical analysis of the exam. In order to discourage wild guessing a heavy penalty is introduced in the form of a negative score for an incorrect answer, which usually results in candidates' answer sheets being returned with a proportion of "don't knows".

The MRCP Part I examination is held three times a year in many centres in the United Kingdom and abroad. A maximum of four attempts at Part I are allowed. Re-entry may be deferred if the candidate fails badly. No set syllabus is published by the Royal Colleges but recently the emphasis of the exam has been on the basic sciences, which will comprise up to 30% of the exam. Sixty multiple choice questions are used from an ever-changing bank of about 4000 questions. A breakdown of the relative distribution of questions is given below.

Topic	No. of questions asked
Anatomy	1
Cardiology	4
Clinical pharmacology	5
Dermatology	1
Endocrinology	3
Gastroenterology	1
Genetics	1
Haematology	2 or 3
Immunology or allergy	1

1

Industrial medicine	1
Infectious diseases	2 or 3
Metabolic disease	2
Musculoskeletal diseases	2
Neurology	4
Ophthalmology	1
Paediatrics	4
Physiology	1
Psychiatry	4
Renal disease	3
Respiratory diseases	4
Reticuloendothelial system	1
Statistics	1
Symptoms and signs	1 or 2
Toxicology	1
Tropical medicine	1 or 0

The exam is essentially competitive, with about the top 30% of candidates passing each time, the passmark therefore being variable. In simple terms, this means that the successful candidate must perform better than the majority of his or her colleagues. Achieving this requires sound knowledge of medicine and basic science, as well as practice in multiple choice question technique.

There is no doubt that at least 12 weeks' serious preparatory work is needed for this exam. A busy clinical job can erode the time spent in the proper preparation which is so necessary for success.

Stage I: This should be a stage of broadly based general reading (see list below), aimed at acquiring good background knowledge.

Stage II: This should be one of using subject-based multiple choice questions to guide detailed reading in areas of weakness. This helps to highlight the fields in which additional reading is valuable. Using multiple choice questions in this way helps the candidate to be guided into those areas on which the College has placed particular emphasis.

Stage III: This stage of preparation for the exam is the most difficult. Many candidates find it hard to take an overall view, but working through multiple choice question papers is probably the best way to polish technique and pick out any final points requiring extra attention. This method also enables one to gain insight into one's own aptitude for multiple choice question exams, which is invaluable when actually sitting the paper. The College quite rightly advises against guessing, but one only learns to assess reasonable certainty by practice and experience.

Bibliography

Bannister R (1985) Brain's clinical neurology, 6th edn. Oxford University Press, Oxford

Burton JL (1983) Aids to postgraduate medicine, 4th edn. Churchill Livingstone, Edinburgh

Ellis H (1983) Clinical anatomy, 7th edn. Blackwell Scientific, Oxford

Forfar JO, Arneil GC (1984) Textbook of paediatrics, vols 1 and 2, 3rd edn. Churchill Livingstone, Edinburgh

Ganong WF (1987) Review of medical physiology, 13th edn. Lange Medical Publications, Los Altos, California

Goodman LS, Gilman A (1985) The pharmacological basis of therapeutics, 7th edn. Macmillan, New York

Isselbacher KJ et al. (eds) (1983) Harrison's principles of internal medicine. McGraw-Hill, New York

Johnson NMcI (1986) Respiratory medicine pocket consultant. Blackwell Scientific, Oxford

Johnson N, Pozniak A (1986) MRCP Part I. Springer, Berlin Heidelberg New York

Patten J (1977) Neurological differential diagnosis. Harold Starke, London

Pocock SJ (1983) Clinical trials: a practical approach. John Wiley & Sons, Chichester

Roitt I et al. (1985) Immunology. Churchill Livingstone, Edinburgh

Rubenstein D, Wayne D (1985) Lecture notes on clinical medicine, 3rd edn. Blackwell Scientific, Oxford

Weatherall DJ (1986) The new genetics and clinical practice, 2nd edn. Oxford University Press, Oxford

Weatherall DJ, Leadingham JGG, Warrell DA (1983) The Oxford textbook of medicine. Oxford University Press, Oxford

Zilva JF, Pannall P (1984) Clinical chemistry in diagnosis and treatment, 4th edn. Lloyd-Luke, London

Examples of Multiple Choice Questions from the Common Part I MRCP (UK), 1st and 2nd series. Royal College of Physicians of Edinburgh, Glasgow and London

Medicine International vols 1 and 2, 1982 onwards, Oxford

Journals: British Medical Journal
British Journal of Hospital Medicine
Hospital Update
The Lancet
New England Journal of Medicine

Addresses of Royal Colleges

Royal College of Physicians of Edinburgh
9 Queen Street
Edinburgh EH2 1JQ

Royal College of Physicians of Glasgow
242 St Vincent Street
Glasgow G2 5RJ

Royal College of Physicians of London
11 St Andrew's Place
Regents Park
London NW1 4LE

How to Use this Book

All of these examination papers have been used in the Bloomsbury MRCP Part I Course which we organise. The passmark given for each paper (with each answer sheet) gives only an arbitrary guide to the performance of previous candidates who have been successful in the membership.

You should use this book as a set of test examinations to be taken in stage III of your revision. By doing so, not only will you gain experience of performing under the stress of a time limit, but you will also be able to assess your strengths and weaknesses. Don't forget to read the questions carefully, check your answers and fill in the answer sheet correctly.

Do these and other questions in your possession over again, coming back repeatedly to those you get wrong.

The Examination

1. You are allowed 2 hours to complete the paper, which is answered on a computer card (see below) with a 2B pencil.

2. Each initial statement or stem has five possible completions, listed (a) to (e).

3. Each of these has to be answered "true", "false" or "don't know" by filling in the appropriate box on the answer sheet.

4. There is no restriction on the number of true or false answers to any question.

Examination 1

All parts of every question must be answered *True* or *False* or *Don't Know* by filling in the box provided. Failure to do so will result in rejection of the answer sheet

SURNAME

INITIALS

Please use 2B PENCIL only. Rub out all errors thoroughly.
Mark lozenges like ▬ NOT like this ⌀ ⌀ ✗

T ⬭ = TRUE   F ⬭ = FALSE   DK ⬭ = DON'T KNOW

	A	B	C	D	E			A	B	C	D	E
1	T / F / DK	T / F / DK	T / F / DK	T / F / DK	T / F / DK		16	T / F / DK	T / F / DK	T / F / DK	T / F / DK	T / F / DK
2	T / F / DK	T / F / DK	T / F / DK	T / F / DK	T / F / DK		17	T / F / DK	T / F / DK	T / F / DK	T / F / DK	T / F / DK
3	T / F / DK	T / F / DK	T / F / DK	T / F / DK	T / F / DK		18	T / F / DK	T / F / DK	T / F / DK	T / F / DK	T / F / DK
4	T / F / DK	T / F / DK	T / F / DK	T / F / DK	T / F / DK		19	T / F / DK	T / F / DK	T / F / DK	T / F / DK	T / F / DK
5	T / F / DK	T / F / DK	T / F / DK	T / F / DK	T / F / DK		20	T / F / DK	T / F / DK	T / F / DK	T / F / DK	T / F / DK
6	T / F / DK	T / F / DK	T / F / DK	T / F / DK	T / F / DK		21	T / F / DK	T / F / DK	T / F / DK	T / F / DK	T / F / DK
7	T / F / DK	T / F / DK	T / F / DK	T / F / DK	T / F / DK		22	T / F / DK	T / F / DK	T / F / DK	T / F / DK	T / F / DK
8	T / F / DK	T / F / DK	T / F / DK	T / F / DK	T / F / DK		23	T / F / DK	T / F / DK	T / F / DK	T / F / DK	T / F / DK
9	T / F / DK	T / F / DK	T / F / DK	T / F / DK	T / F / DK		24	T / F / DK	T / F / DK	T / F / DK	T / F / DK	T / F / DK
10	T / F / DK	T / F / DK	T / F / DK	T / F / DK	T / F / DK		25	T / F / DK	T / F / DK	T / F / DK	T / F / DK	T / F / DK
11	T / F / DK	T / F / DK	T / F / DK	T / F / DK	T / F / DK		26	T / F / DK	T / F / DK	T / F / DK	T / F / DK	T / F / DK
12	T / F / DK	T / F / DK	T / F / DK	T / F / DK	T / F / DK		27	T / F / DK	T / F / DK	T / F / DK	T / F / DK	T / F / DK
13	T / F / DK	T / F / DK	T / F / DK	T / F / DK	T / F / DK		28	T / F / DK	T / F / DK	T / F / DK	T / F / DK	T / F / DK
14	T / F / DK	T / F / DK	T / F / DK	T / F / DK	T / F / DK		29	T / F / DK	T / F / DK	T / F / DK	T / F / DK	T / F / DK
15	T / F / DK	T / F / DK	T / F / DK	T / F / DK	T / F / DK		30	T / F / DK	T / F / DK	T / F / DK	T / F / DK	T / F / DK

	A	B	C	D	E		A	B	C	D	E
31	T F DK	T F DK	T F DK	T F DK	T F DK	**46**	T F DK	T F DK	T F DK	T F DK	T F DK
32	T F DK	T F DK	T F DK	T F DK	T F DK	**47**	T F DK	T F DK	T F DK	T F DK	T F DK
33	T F DK	T F DK	T F DK	T F DK	T F DK	**48**	T F DK	T F DK	T F DK	T F DK	T F DK
34	T F DK	T F DK	T F DK	T F DK	T F DK	**49**	T F DK	T F DK	T F DK	T F DK	T F DK
35	T F DK	T F DK	T F DK	T F DK	T F DK	**50**	T F DK	T F DK	T F DK	T F DK	T F DK
36	T F DK	T F DK	T F DK	T F DK	T F DK	**51**	T F DK	T F DK	T F DK	T F DK	T F DK
37	T F DK	T F DK	T F DK	T F DK	T F DK	**52**	T F DK	T F DK	T F DK	T F DK	T F DK
38	T F DK	T F DK	T F DK	T F DK	T F DK	**53**	T F DK	T F DK	T F DK	T F DK	T F DK
39	T F DK	T F DK	T F DK	T F DK	T F DK	**54**	T F DK	T F DK	T F DK	T F DK	T F DK
40	T F DK	T F DK	T F DK	T F DK	T F DK	**55**	T F DK	T F DK	T F DK	T F DK	T F DK
41	T F DK	T F DK	T F DK	T F DK	T F DK	**56**	T F DK	T F DK	T F DK	T F DK	T F DK
42	T F DK	T F DK	T F DK	T F DK	T F DK	**57**	T F DK	T F DK	T F DK	T F DK	T F DK
43	T F DK	T F DK	T F DK	T F DK	T F DK	**58**	T F DK	T F DK	T F DK	T F DK	T F DK
44	T F DK	T F DK	T F DK	T F DK	T F DK	**59**	T F DK	T F DK	T F DK	T F DK	T F DK
45	T F DK	T F DK	T F DK	T F DK	T F DK	**60**	T F DK	T F DK	T F DK	T F DK	T F DK

1. Which of the following anatomical statements are true?

   a) The maxillary division of the trigeminal nerve traverses the skull through the foramen rotundum
   b) The angle of the jaw is innervated by the mandibular division of the trigeminal nerve
   c) The glossopharyngeal nerve is motor to the palate
   d) The chorda tympani joins the facial nerve at the geniculate ganglion
   e) The arteria magna of Adamkiewicz is a branch of a lower thoracic intercostal artery

2. Which of the following are indications of acute left ventricular failure?

   a) Elevated pCO_2
   b) Tachycardia
   c) Normal left ventricular end-diastolic pressure
   d) Ankle oedema
   e) Third heart sound

3. Which of the following may be indications for nifedipine therapy?

   a) Mild heart failure
   b) Polyarteritis nodosa
   c) Prinzmetal's angina
   d) Intermittent claudication
   e) Raynaud's disease

4. Which of the following are common features of coarctation of the aorta?

   a) Neonatal hypertension
   b) Ebstein's anomaly
   c) Treatment with balloon angioplasty
   d) Dilatation of the pulmonary arteries
   e) Biscuspid aortic valve

5. Which of the following features may occur in association with tricuspid regurgitation?

   a) Multiple pulmonary abscesses
   b) Pulsatile spleen
   c) Distinctive appearances on echocardiography
   d) Giant "a" venous wave
   e) Ankle oedema

6. Which of the following drugs are implicated in acute renal failure due to tubular necrosis?

   a) Tetracyclines
   b) Phenacetin
   c) Naproxen
   d) Sulphonamides
   e) Cyclosporin

7. Which of the following are side-effects of penicillamine?

   a) Mammary hyperplasia
   b) Goodpasture's syndrome
   c) Lupus erythematosus syndrome
   d) Loss of taste
   e) Hepatitis

8. Which of the following factors may precipitate hepatic encephalopathy?

   a) Laxatives
   b) Urinary infection
   c) Prolonged fast
   d) Diazepam
   e) Diuretics

9. Plasma exchange:

   a) Is the same as plasmapheresis
   b) May be of benefit in Guillain–Barré syndrome
   c) Consists of removing less than 1 litre of plasma and replacing it with colloid
   d) Is not effective in motor neurone disease
   e) Is rarely associated with complications

10. Which of the following may precipitate or worsen psoriasis?

   a) Streptococcal sore throat
   b) Lithium
   c) Hydroxyurea
   d) Sunlight
   e) Antimalarials

11. Cutaneous calcinosis may occur in:

   a) Pseudoxanthoma elasticum
   b) Dermatomyositis
   c) Syphilis
   d) Scleroderma
   e) Sarcoid

12. Hirsutism may result from:

   a) Minoxidil
   b) Prednisone
   c) Empty sella syndrome
   d) Polycystic ovary syndrome
   e) Radiotherapy

13. Vasopressin release is inhibited by:

   a) Hypoalbuminaemia
   b) Hypoxaemia
   c) Nicotine
   d) Coitus
   e) Carbamazepine

14. Hypopituitarism may result from:

   a) Somatostatin treatment
   b) Steroid therapy
   c) Syphilis
   d) Sarcoidosis
   e) Isoniazid

15. In which situations is the hyperbilirubinaemia predominantly conjugated?

   a) Crigler–Najjar syndrome
   b) Rotor's syndrome
   c) Dubin–Johnson syndrome
   d) Caroli's syndrome
   e) Gilbert's syndrome

16. Which of the following features suggest a diagnosis of Crohn's disease rather than ulcerative colitis?

    a) Transmural inflammation
    b) Abdominal mass
    c) Crypt abscesses
    d) Fistula
    e) Cobblestoning

17. Adenocarcinoma of the stomach is associated with:

    a) Pernicious anaemia
    b) Acanthosis nigricans
    c) Diarrhoea
    d) Chronic iron deficiency
    e) Blood group O

18. Which of the following statements are true?

    a) Hereditary angioedema is caused by C_1 esterase inhibitor deficiency
    b) The exon is the gene segment encoding protein
    c) Hybridomas are cell lines from a single cell type
    d) Epitope combines with paratope
    e) High endothelial venules are common in the liver

19. In "the new genetics":

    a) cDNA stands for cloned DNA
    b) Southern blotting refers to the transfer of DNA segments from nitrocellulose filters to agarose electrophoresis columns
    c) cDNA is made from mRNA by reverse transcriptase
    d) Restriction fragment length polymorphisms are inherited in a Mendelian fashion
    e) cDNA duplexes may be cloned in bacterial plasmids

20. Hypochromic anaemia may result from:

    a) Thalassaemia
    b) Sickle cell disease
    c) Lead poisoning
    d) Hereditary spherocytosis
    e) Pregnancy

21. Neutropenia may result from:
    a) Acute haemorrhage
    b) Warm autoimmune haemolytic anaemia
    c) Ranitidine
    d) Corticosteroids
    e) Metastatic cancer

22. In Hodgkin's disease:
    a) Development of a second malignancy is a common complication of treatment
    b) There is often a high titre of antibodies to the Epstein–Barr virus
    c) The current 5-year survival is 50%
    d) The skin is frequently involved with lymphoma
    e) The prognosis is affected by the presence of systemic features at presentation

23. Interleukin-2 is:
    a) Secreted by T lymphocytes
    b) Augmented by γ-interferon
    c) A lymphokine
    d) Secreted by macrophages
    e) An inhibitor of T cell proliferation

24. Which of the following statements are true?
    a) Class 2 (HLA DR) antigens are complement components encoded by the major histocompatibility complex
    b) The mixed lymphocyte reaction depends on the ability of lymphocytes to proliferate on recognition of foreign HLA specificities on typing lymphocytes
    c) Monoclonal antibodies are produced by immunising an animal with the chosen antigen and then fusing its spleen cells with those of an immortal non-secretor myeloma line
    d) Allotypic variation refers to the antigenic characteristics of the hypervariable region of the immunoglobulin molecule
    e) Leukotrienes are a group of peptides that signal between cells of the immune system

25. Patients with which of the following asbestos-related diseases are eligible for compensation under DHSS regulations?

   a) Bronchial carcinoma
   b) Pleural thickening (benign)
   c) Asbestosis
   d) Mesothelioma
   e) Asthma

26. In HIV disease:

   a) Anoreceptive homosexual males are at the greatest risk of infection
   b) The virus selectively infects T suppressor cells
   c) Kaposi's sarcoma carries a worse prognosis in AIDS than *Pneumocystis carinii* pneumonia
   d) AIDS is notifiable
   e) Regression of the lymphadenopathy in progressive generalised lymphadenopathy indicates reversion to the asymptomatic carrier state

27. Which of the following statements are true of hepatitis B but not of hepatitis A?

   a) It is a notifiable disease to the Medical Officer of Health
   b) Chronic liver disease is a recognised complication
   c) Transmission does not occur by the faeco-oral route
   d) Passive immunity can be acquired from pooled gamma globulin
   e) Alcohol should be avoided for 1 year after recovery

28. In cases of whooping cough:

   a) The child may appear to be completely well
   b) The diagnosis is supported by finding a lymphopenia
   c) Babies under the age of 6 months are not at risk
   d) Erythromycin is the antibiotic of choice
   e) The disease is notifiable to the Medical Officer of Health

29. Which of the following associations of specific enzyme deficiency are correct?

a) Tangier disease – beta-lipoproteinase
b) Fabry's disease – sphingomyelinase
c) Gaucher's disease – galactosidase A
d) Tay–Sachs disease – glucoserebrosidase
e) Niemann–Pick disease – hexosaminodase A

30. In diabetes mellitus:

a) The chance of retinopathy is not significantly related to the duration of diabetes
b) Clinical proteinuria (>0.5 g/day) means end-stage renal failure in under 5 years
c) Proliferative retinopathy is associated with the development of new vessels on the anterior surface of the iris
d) Most patients presenting with diabetic ketoacidosis are previously undiagnosed diabetics
e) Hospital admission is indicated for all cases of hypoglycaemia due to sulphonylureas

31. Which of the following are features of Paget's disease?

a) Prominent scalp veins
b) Nocturnal pain
c) Proximal muscle weakness
d) Inclusion bodies in the abnormal large multinuclear osteoclasts
e) Decreased 24-hour urinary hydroxyproline excretion

32. Which of the following are radiological features of rheumatoid arthritis?

a) Bone cysts
b) Resorption of the distal ends of the clavicles
c) Erosions at the joint margins
d) Juxta-articular osteoporosis
e) Osteophyte formation

33. In head injury:

   a) The severity is related to the period of anterograde amnesia
   b) Concussion is associated with structural brain damage
   c) A hemiplegia is a useful lateralising sign
   d) The blood gases of an unconscious patient should always be measured
   e) The Glasgow Coma Scale is based on assessment of the best verbal response, the best motor response and the response to painful stimuli

34. In multiple sclerosis:

   a) The prevalence is high in the tropics
   b) Sites of predilection are the cervical cord, the brain stem and cortical periventricular structures
   c) Thirty per cent of patients progress without remission
   d) The CSF protein is reduced
   e) Significant sensory symptoms are often dismissed as hysterical

35. In Parkinson's disease:

   a) Patients have often been heavy smokers
   b) Deprenyl is a specific monoamine oxidase B inhibitor
   c) A high-protein diet may interfere with the therapeutic effect of L-dopa
   d) Over the age of 60 the prevalence is 1 in 100
   e) Seborrhoea is common

36. In migraine:

   a) It is necessary to have an aura to make the diagnosis
   b) Pregnancy is usually associated with a worsening of the severity
   c) There is an association with cerebral angioma
   d) Drug absorption is increased
   e) The headache is usually unilateral

37. In which of the following conditions is the pulmonary wedge pressure increased?

   a) Uncomplicated myocardial infarction
   b) Mitral stenosis
   c) Pulmonary embolism
   d) Right ventricular infarct
   e) Cardiogenic shock

38. The serum alkaline phosphatase is often normal in:

   a) Cirrhosis
   b) Gilbert's disease
   c) Viral hepatitis
   d) Amoebic liver abscess
   e) Multiple myeloma

39. In paediatric oncology:

   a) Neuroblastoma may regress spontaneously
   b) Nephroblastoma is frequently bilateral
   c) Histiocytosis X may present with polydipsia
   d) Solid tumours are commoner than leukaemia
   e) The commonest posterior fossa tumour is a craniopharyngioma

40. In infectious mononucleosis:

   a) The cause of the illness is a herpes virus
   b) Infected lymphocytes appear in the peripheral circulation as atypical mononuclear cells
   c) Jaundice is common
   d) The administration of corticosteroids may precipitate polyneuritis or thrombocytopenia
   e) Previous injection of horse anti-tetanus serum gives a false positive Paul–Bunnell test

41. Complications of diabetic pregnancy include:

   a) Pre-eclampsia
   b) Neonatal hypoglycaemia
   c) Hydramnios
   d) High HbA1c
   e) Fetal macrosomy

42. Fresh frozen plasma:

    a) Is free of risk of infection
    b) One unit should be given routinely with every 4 units of stored blood
    c) Should be given to all patients with liver disease before needle biopsy
    d) Is a by-product of the manufacture of factor VIII
    e) Is indicated for the treatment of factor V deficiency

43. Causes of hypernatraemia include:

    a) Bartter's syndrome
    b) Cushing's disease
    c) Acute renal failure
    d) Diabetes mellitus
    e) Diabetes insipidus

44. Deliberate self-harm:

    a) Is usually associated with recent alcohol intake
    b) Is often associated with florid psychosis
    c) Is frequently followed by completed suicide
    d) May constitute as many as 20% of all acute admissions to hospital in the UK
    e) Commonly follows difficulties with inter-personal relationships

45. In the elderly:

    a) There is a second peak in the incidence of dermatitis herpetiformis
    b) With an attack of shingles there is a good chance of there being an underlying malignancy
    c) Erythroplasia of Queyrat is a benign lymphocytic balanitis
    d) Lentigo maligna melanoma is the commonest facial malignancy
    e) Morphoeic basal cell carcinoma is the most radio-sensitive carcinoma

46. In classical distal renal tubular acidosis:

    a) The urinary bicarbonate is increased
    b) The serum potassium is elevated
    c) The urinary pH is greater than 5.5 after an acid load
    d) The net acid excretion is normal
    e) Weight loss greater than 3 kg after 12 hours of fluid
       deprivation aids diagnosis

47. Renal glycosuria may be associated with:

    a) A normal blood glucose
    b) Medullary sponge kidney
    c) Cystinuria
    d) Autosomal dominant inheritance
    e) Increased risk of diabetes mellitus

48. In acute renal failure:

    a) The diagnosis depends upon anuria or oliguria (<15 ml/
       hour)
    b) The aetiology is often multifactorial
    c) Eosinophilia may suggest that a drug is the cause
    d) Hyperkalaemia (e.g. >7 mmol/l) should be treated
       urgently
    e) Attention to the nutritional status is a high priority in
       the early stages

49. Regarding the assessment of renal function:

    a) Inulin clearance is the most clinically useful measure of
       glomerular filtration rate
    b) The glomerular filtration rate varies inversely with the
       plasma creatinine concentration
    c) Urine osmolality is measured by observing how much the
       freezing point is depressed
    d) With a plasma bicarbonate <20 mmol/l, the urinary pH
       should be > 5.3
    e) A disproportionately high plasma creatinine
       concentration may be found in patients taking
       tetracyclines

50. Which of the following are associated with small (oat) cell carcinoma of the bronchus?

   a) Hypertrophic pulmonary osteoarthropathy
   b) Hypercalcaemia
   c) Gynaecomastia
   d) Inappropriate ADH secretion
   e) Cushing's syndrome

51. Pulmonary fibrosis may be caused by:

   a) Radiotherapy
   b) Gallium
   c) Aspirin
   d) Bleomycin
   e) Heroin

52. The arterial pCO_2 is typically raised in:

   a) Respiratory failure secondary to pneumonia
   b) Sleep apnoea
   c) Mild asthma attack
   d) Renal failure
   e) Anorexia nervosa

53. Cor pulmonale can be associated with:

   a) Schistosomiasis
   b) Myasthenia gravis
   c) Asthma
   d) Sleep apnoea syndrome
   e) Pulmonary emboli

54. Which of the following are complications of chronic lymphatic leukaemia?

   a) Monoclonal gammopathy
   b) Autoimmune thrombocytopenia
   c) Autoimmune haemolytic anaemia
   d) Hypogammaglobulinaemia
   e) Priapism

55. The mean corpuscular volume is high in:

   a) Thalassaemia
   b) Aplastic anaemia
   c) Thyrotoxicosis
   d) The anaemia of chronic renal failure
   e) Haemolysis

56. Familial hypercholesterolaemia:

   a) Is an autosomal recessive condition
   b) Is associated with markedly elevated triglyceride levels
   c) Results from a genetic deficiency of low-density
      lipoproteins
   d) Is not associated with improved mortality and morbidity
      when treated
   e) Is associated with eruptive xanthomata, lipaemia retinalis
      and acute pancreatitis

57. Which of the following are signs of portal hypertension?

   a) Spider naevi
   b) Hepatomegaly
   c) Venous hum
   d) Ascites
   e) Caput medusae

58. Which of the following antidotes are linked with the
    appropriate poison/drug:

   a) Pralidoxime mesylate – malathion
   b) Dicobalt edetate – mercury
   c) Prenalterol – sotalol
   d) Fab antibody fragments – digoxin
   e) Dimercaprol – arsenic

59. Pre-hepatic portal hypertension may result from:

   a) Sarcoidosis
   b) Splenomegaly
   c) Portal vein thrombosis
   d) Schistosomiasis
   e) Budd–Chiari syndrome

60. Which of the following statements about sexually transmitted diseases are true?

a) Herpes simplex virus (type 1) does not cause genital herpes
b) Generalised complications of gonorrhoea are more common in women
c) There is no completely specific serological test for syphilis
d) γ-Benzene hexachloride is preferred to benzyl benzoate for the treatment of infestations in pregnancy
e) Having a partner with penile condylomata acuminata is a risk factor for cervical cancer

Examination 2

All parts of every question must
be answered *True* or *False* or
Don't Know by filling in the box
provided. Failure to do so will
result in rejection of the
answer sheet

EXAMINATION NO.

2

SURNAME

INITIALS

Please use 2B PENCIL only. Rub out all errors thoroughly.
Mark lozenges like ● NOT like this ⌀ ⌀ ✗

T ⌷ = **TRUE**   F ⌷ = **FALSE**   DK ⌷ = **DON'T KNOW**

	A	B	C	D	E			A	B	C	D	E
1	T / F / DK	T / F / DK	T / F / DK	T / F / DK	T / F / DK		16	T / F / DK	T / F / DK	T / F / DK	T / F / DK	T / F / DK
2	T / F / DK	T / F / DK	T / F / DK	T / F / DK	T / F / DK		17	T / F / DK	T / F / DK	T / F / DK	T / F / DK	T / F / DK
3	T / F / DK	T / F / DK	T / F / DK	T / F / DK	T / F / DK		18	T / F / DK	T / F / DK	T / F / DK	T / F / DK	T / F / DK
4	T / F / DK	T / F / DK	T / F / DK	T / F / DK	T / F / DK		19	T / F / DK	T / F / DK	T / F / DK	T / F / DK	T / F / DK
5	T / F / DK	T / F / DK	T / F / DK	T / F / DK	T / F / DK		20	T / F / DK	T / F / DK	T / F / DK	T / F / DK	T / F / DK
6	T / F / DK	T / F / DK	T / F / DK	T / F / DK	T / F / DK		21	T / F / DK	T / F / DK	T / F / DK	T / F / DK	T / F / DK
7	T / F / DK	T / F / DK	T / F / DK	T / F / DK	T / F / DK		22	T / F / DK	T / F / DK	T / F / DK	T / F / DK	T / F / DK
8	T / F / DK	T / F / DK	T / F / DK	T / F / DK	T / F / DK		23	T / F / DK	T / F / DK	T / F / DK	T / F / DK	T / F / DK
9	T / F / DK	T / F / DK	T / F / DK	T / F / DK	T / F / DK		24	T / F / DK	T / F / DK	T / F / DK	T / F / DK	T / F / DK
10	T / F / DK	T / F / DK	T / F / DK	T / F / DK	T / F / DK		25	T / F / DK	T / F / DK	T / F / DK	T / F / DK	T / F / DK
11	T / F / DK	T / F / DK	T / F / DK	T / F / DK	T / F / DK		26	T / F / DK	T / F / DK	T / F / DK	T / F / DK	T / F / DK
12	T / F / DK	T / F / DK	T / F / DK	T / F / DK	T / F / DK		27	T / F / DK	T / F / DK	T / F / DK	T / F / DK	T / F / DK
13	T / F / DK	T / F / DK	T / F / DK	T / F / DK	T / F / DK		28	T / F / DK	T / F / DK	T / F / DK	T / F / DK	T / F / DK
14	T / F / DK	T / F / DK	T / F / DK	T / F / DK	T / F / DK		29	T / F / DK	T / F / DK	T / F / DK	T / F / DK	T / F / DK
15	T / F / DK	T / F / DK	T / F / DK	T / F / DK	T / F / DK		30	T / F / DK	T / F / DK	T / F / DK	T / F / DK	T / F / DK

	A	B	C	D	E			A	B	C	D	E
31	T ⬭	T ⬭	T ⬭	T ⬭	T ⬭		46	T ⬭	T ⬭	T ⬭	T ⬭	T ⬭
	F ⬭	F ⬭	F ⬭	F ⬭	F ⬭			F ⬭	F ⬭	F ⬭	F ⬭	F ⬭
	DK ⬭	DK ⬭	DK ⬭	DK ⬭	DK ⬭			DK ⬭	DK ⬭	DK ⬭	DK ⬭	DK ⬭
32	T ⬭	T ⬭	T ⬭	T ⬭	T ⬭		47	T ⬭	T ⬭	T ⬭	T ⬭	T ⬭
	F ⬭	F ⬭	F ⬭	F ⬭	F ⬭			F ⬭	F ⬭	F ⬭	F ⬭	F ⬭
	DK ⬭	DK ⬭	DK ⬭	DK ⬭	DK ⬭			DK ⬭	DK ⬭	DK ⬭	DK ⬭	DK ⬭
33	T ⬭	T ⬭	T ⬭	T ⬭	T ⬭		48	T ⬭	T ⬭	T ⬭	T ⬭	T ⬭
	F ⬭	F ⬭	F ⬭	F ⬭	F ⬭			F ⬭	F ⬭	F ⬭	F ⬭	F ⬭
	DK ⬭	DK ⬭	DK ⬭	DK ⬭	DK ⬭			DK ⬭	DK ⬭	DK ⬭	DK ⬭	DK ⬭
34	T ⬭	T ⬭	T ⬭	T ⬭	T ⬭		49	T ⬭	T ⬭	T ⬭	T ⬭	T ⬭
	F ⬭	F ⬭	F ⬭	F ⬭	F ⬭			F ⬭	F ⬭	F ⬭	F ⬭	F ⬭
	DK ⬭	DK ⬭	DK ⬭	DK ⬭	DK ⬭			DK ⬭	DK ⬭	DK ⬭	DK ⬭	DK ⬭
35	T ⬭	T ⬭	T ⬭	T ⬭	T ⬭		50	T ⬭	T ⬭	T ⬭	T ⬭	T ⬭
	F ⬭	F ⬭	F ⬭	F ⬭	F ⬭			F ⬭	F ⬭	F ⬭	F ⬭	F ⬭
	DK ⬭	DK ⬭	DK ⬭	DK ⬭	DK ⬭			DK ⬭	DK ⬭	DK ⬭	DK ⬭	DK ⬭
36	T ⬭	T ⬭	T ⬭	T ⬭	T ⬭		51	T ⬭	T ⬭	T ⬭	T ⬭	T ⬭
	F ⬭	F ⬭	F ⬭	F ⬭	F ⬭			F ⬭	F ⬭	F ⬭	F ⬭	F ⬭
	DK ⬭	DK ⬭	DK ⬭	DK ⬭	DK ⬭			DK ⬭	DK ⬭	DK ⬭	DK ⬭	DK ⬭
37	T ⬭	T ⬭	T ⬭	T ⬭	T ⬭		52	T ⬭	T ⬭	T ⬭	T ⬭	T ⬭
	F ⬭	F ⬭	F ⬭	F ⬭	F ⬭			F ⬭	F ⬭	F ⬭	F ⬭	F ⬭
	DK ⬭	DK ⬭	DK ⬭	DK ⬭	DK ⬭			DK ⬭	DK ⬭	DK ⬭	DK ⬭	DK ⬭
38	T ⬭	T ⬭	T ⬭	T ⬭	T ⬭		53	T ⬭	T ⬭	T ⬭	T ⬭	T ⬭
	F ⬭	F ⬭	F ⬭	F ⬭	F ⬭			F ⬭	F ⬭	F ⬭	F ⬭	F ⬭
	DK ⬭	DK ⬭	DK ⬭	DK ⬭	DK ⬭			DK ⬭	DK ⬭	DK ⬭	DK ⬭	DK ⬭
39	T ⬭	T ⬭	T ⬭	T ⬭	T ⬭		54	T ⬭	T ⬭	T ⬭	T ⬭	T ⬭
	F ⬭	F ⬭	F ⬭	F ⬭	F ⬭			F ⬭	F ⬭	F ⬭	F ⬭	F ⬭
	DK ⬭	DK ⬭	DK ⬭	DK ⬭	DK ⬭			DK ⬭	DK ⬭	DK ⬭	DK ⬭	DK ⬭
40	T ⬭	T ⬭	T ⬭	T ⬭	T ⬭		55	T ⬭	T ⬭	T ⬭	T ⬭	T ⬭
	F ⬭	F ⬭	F ⬭	F ⬭	F ⬭			F ⬭	F ⬭	F ⬭	F ⬭	F ⬭
	DK ⬭	DK ⬭	DK ⬭	DK ⬭	DK ⬭			DK ⬭	DK ⬭	DK ⬭	DK ⬭	DK ⬭
41	T ⬭	T ⬭	T ⬭	T ⬭	T ⬭		56	T ⬭	T ⬭	T ⬭	T ⬭	T ⬭
	F ⬭	F ⬭	F ⬭	F ⬭	F ⬭			F ⬭	F ⬭	F ⬭	F ⬭	F ⬭
	DK ⬭	DK ⬭	DK ⬭	DK ⬭	DK ⬭			DK ⬭	DK ⬭	DK ⬭	DK ⬭	DK ⬭
42	T ⬭	T ⬭	T ⬭	T ⬭	T ⬭		57	T ⬭	T ⬭	T ⬭	T ⬭	T ⬭
	F ⬭	F ⬭	F ⬭	F ⬭	F ⬭			F ⬭	F ⬭	F ⬭	F ⬭	F ⬭
	DK ⬭	DK ⬭	DK ⬭	DK ⬭	DK ⬭			DK ⬭	DK ⬭	DK ⬭	DK ⬭	DK ⬭
43	T ⬭	T ⬭	T ⬭	T ⬭	T ⬭		58	T ⬭	T ⬭	T ⬭	T ⬭	T ⬭
	F ⬭	F ⬭	F ⬭	F ⬭	F ⬭			F ⬭	F ⬭	F ⬭	F ⬭	F ⬭
	DK ⬭	DK ⬭	DK ⬭	DK ⬭	DK ⬭			DK ⬭	DK ⬭	DK ⬭	DK ⬭	DK ⬭
44	T ⬭	T ⬭	T ⬭	T ⬭	T ⬭		59	T ⬭	T ⬭	T ⬭	T ⬭	T ⬭
	F ⬭	F ⬭	F ⬭	F ⬭	F ⬭			F ⬭	F ⬭	F ⬭	F ⬭	F ⬭
	DK ⬭	DK ⬭	DK ⬭	DK ⬭	DK ⬭			DK ⬭	DK ⬭	DK ⬭	DK ⬭	DK ⬭
45	T ⬭	T ⬭	T ⬭	T ⬭	T ⬭		60	T ⬭	T ⬭	T ⬭	T ⬭	T ⬭
	F ⬭	F ⬭	F ⬭	F ⬭	F ⬭			F ⬭	F ⬭	F ⬭	F ⬭	F ⬭
	DK ⬭	DK ⬭	DK ⬭	DK ⬭	DK ⬭			DK ⬭	DK ⬭	DK ⬭	DK ⬭	DK ⬭

1. Which of the following statements about the lung are true?

   a) The cross-sectional area of the alveolar capillary membrane is approximately 1000 m^2
   b) The lingula is part of the upper lobe of the left lung
   c) Blood flow is greatest in the upper lobes
   d) Surfactant is produced by type II pneumocytes
   e) Compliance is increased in pulmonary oedema

2. Which of the following statements concerning artificial heart valves are true?

   a) Aortic valves are more likely to be sources of emboli than mitral valves
   b) Residual gradients occur across replaced valves
   c) Antibiotic cover is required for genitourinary surgery
   d) Anticoagulation is not required with a Starr–Edwards valve
   e) Haemolytic anaemia may be caused by normally functioning valves

3. Which of the following are major criteria (Jones criteria) for the diagnosis of rheumatic fever?

   a) Fever
   b) Chorea
   c) Prolonged PR interval
   d) Erythema marginatum
   e) Raised antistreptolysin O titre

4. Which of the following are side-effects of or contraindications to beta-blocker therapy?

   a) Parkinson's disease
   b) Asthma
   c) Wolff–Parkinson–White syndrome
   d) Atrial fibrillation due to thyrotoxicosis
   e) Raynaud's syndrome

5. Regarding the prognosis of myocardial infarction:
   a) It can be reliably assessed by early exercise ECG testing
   b) Approximately 15% of resuscitations in hospital are successful
   c) It is not related to the amount of heart muscle damaged
   d) Twenty-five per cent of patients die immediately
   e) Most of the patients who survive to leave hospital are alive at 1 year

6. Which of the following increase the clearance of ingested theophyllines from the body?
   a) Oral contraceptives
   b) Marijuana smoking
   c) Phenytoin
   d) Cirrhosis of the liver
   e) Cigarette smoking

7. In pharmacokinetics and pharmacodynamics:
   a) The potency of a drug is defined by the position of its log dose–response curve along the horizontal (x) axis
   b) Saturation kinetics refer to the change from zero-order to first-order kinetics when a metabolic pathway is saturated
   c) The volume of distribution (Vd) is the dose of a drug divided by the concentration at time zero (C_0)
   d) Bioavailability describes the fraction of an oral dose of a drug that becomes available for absorption
   e) Pharmacodynamics is the study of the time course of a drug's absorption, distribution, metabolism and excretion

8. Retinoids:
   a) Have side-effects corresponding to the hypervitaminosis E syndrome
   b) Interfere with thyroid function
   c) Contraindicate blood donation
   d) Have anti-neoplastic potential
   e) Are not available outside the hospital clinic

9. Regarding drug information and monitoring:

 a) The BNF is revised every year
 b) The Data Sheet Compendium is published independently of the pharmaceutical industry
 c) There is a fee payable on receipt of a completed "yellow card" by the CSM
 d) Information on poisons is available by telephone from several centres in the UK on a 24-hour basis
 e) A pharmaceutical company has a statutory duty to undertake post-marketing surveillance of its products

10. Genetic polymorphisms influence the metabolism of the following drugs:

 a) Sulphapyridine
 b) Suxamethonium
 c) Isoniazid
 d) Nortriptyline
 e) Hydralazine

11. The Mental Health Act:

 a) Was passed in 1983
 b) Allows a qualified nurse to hold a patient in hospital for 3 days under section 5
 c) Allows two doctors to detain a patient for treatment for 6 months under section 3
 d) Allows a police constable to remove a patient from a public place for medical examination under section 136
 e) Is kept under review by the Mental Health Commission

12. In thyroid crisis:

 a) There may be a precipitating infection
 b) There is almost invariably fever
 c) The benefit of steroids has been ascertained
 d) It is crucial to demonstrate a diminished or absent response of thyrotropin to thyrotropin-releasing hormone
 e) There may be hepatomegaly

13. Which of the following are physiological causes of hyperprolactinaemia in women?

    a) Puberty
    b) Pregnancy
    c) Orgasm
    d) Chlorpromazine
    e) Suckling

14. In the hypercalcaemia of malignancy:

    a) Indomethacin may be beneficial
    b) Improvement can be elicited with a thiazide diuretic
    c) Tamoxifen is always beneficial in cases due to breast disease
    d) Correction of dehydration is the most significant therapeutic measure
    e) There may not be evidence of skeletal metastases

15. Diarrhoea in association with arthritis may be caused by:

    a) Sarcoidosis
    b) Ulcerative colitis
    c) Gonorrhoea
    d) Osler–Weber–Rendu syndrome
    e) Whipple's disease

16. Which of the following may cause malabsorption?

    a) Hodgkin's disease
    b) Ulcerative colitis
    c) Amyloidosis
    d) Gastrinoma
    e) Anorexia nervosa

17. Which of the following typically cause food poisoning within 30 minutes?

    a) Mushroom poisoning
    b) Staphylococcal toxin
    c) Paralytic shellfish poisoning
    d) Chinese restaurant syndrome
    e) Scombroid fish poisoning

18. Which of the following statements about genetics are true?

    a) Half the sons of a mating receive their father's X chromosome
    b) The chromosome number doubles before the first reduction division of meiosis
    c) In DNA uracil pairs with thymine
    d) An autosomal recessive trait is suggested by a condition that affects brothers and sisters with normal parents
    e) Functional coding sequences of genes are called introns

19. Which of the following are phases of the normal cell cycle?

    a) G_2
    b) L
    c) N
    d) T
    e) K

20. A neutrophil leucocytosis may result from:

    a) Acute haemolysis
    b) HIV infection
    c) Hypersplenism
    d) Felty's syndrome
    e) Co-trimoxazole

21. Which of the following may be associated with polycythaemia rubra vera?

    a) Tinnitus
    b) Thrombocytopenia
    c) Itching
    d) Gout
    e) Congestive cardiac failure

22. Which of the following are common presenting features in Hodgkin's disease?

    a) Alcohol-induced pain in lymph nodes
    b) Pel–Ebstein fever
    c) Skeletal involvement
    d) Cervical lymphadenopathy
    e) Intracranial space-occupying lesion

23. Fc cell surface receptors may occur on:

   a) Mast cells
   b) Alveolar macrophages
   c) B lymphocytes
   d) Basophils
   e) Eosinophils

24. Circulating immune complexes have been described in:

   a) Polyarteritis
   b) Bacterial endocarditis
   c) Tuberculosis
   d) Malaria
   e) Fibrosing alveolitis

25. Which of the following occupational carcinogens are correctly linked with their associated neoplasm?

   a) Vinyl chloride – angiosarcoma of the liver
   b) Soot – cancer of the scrotum
   c) Crocodilite – mesothelioma
   d) β-Naphthylamine – bladder cancer
   e) Nickel – nasal sinus cancer

26. The mucocutaneous manifestations of HIV infection include:

   a) *Pityrosporum* folliculitis
   b) Hairy leucoplakia
   c) Seborrhoeic dermatitis
   d) Molluscum contagiosum
   e) Tinea pedis

27. In cases of mumps:

   a) Orchitis rarely leads to infertility
   b) The finding of a raised serum amylase suggests the development of pancreatitis
   c) With involvement of the eighth cranial nerve, balance is usually more severely affected than hearing
   d) Aseptic meningitis is the commonest neurological complication
   e) Presternal oedema is a sign of submandibular gland involvement

28. In rheumatic fever:

 a) Post-streptococcal glomerulonephritis and rheumatic fever rarely follow the same streptococcal infection
 b) One attack increases many-fold the risk of subsequent attacks
 c) Chorea, erythema marginatum and carditis are all attributable to the same type of pathological lesion
 d) It is necessary to demonstrate a fourfold increase in antistreptolysin O or anti-DNAse titre to establish evidence of a recent streptococcal infection
 e) Mitral stenosis is the commonest valvular lesion

29. Regarding the porphyrias:

 a) Congenital erythropoietic porphyria is inherited as an autosomal dominant disorder
 b) Cyclopropane and suxamethonium are regarded as a safe anaesthetic combination for the porphyric patient
 c) A pointer to the need for ventilation in an acute attack is progressive weakness of the voice
 d) A low carbohydrate intake is an essential part of the management of both prophylaxis and an acute attack
 e) Permanent deformity can result from an acute attack

30. In diabetes mellitus:

 a) Few newly diagnosed insulin-dependent diabetics have islet cell surface antibodies
 b) Non-insulin-dependent diabetes is associated with HLA DR3 and DR4
 c) Euglycaemic "clamping" in vivo shows decreased insulin sensitivity in non-insulin-dependent diabetes
 d) Lipoatrophy is an immune-related problem of insulin therapy
 e) High-fibre diets improve glycaemic control solely by reducing the amount of calories consumed as fat

31. Rheumatoid factor:

 a) May be IgM, IgG or IgA
 b) Is fundamental to the aetiology of rheumatoid arthritis
 c) Is always directed against IgG
 d) May be found in cryoproteinaemia
 e) Is absent in about 30% of patients with rheumatoid arthritis

32. Sjögren's syndrome may be associated with:

a) Rheumatoid arthritis
b) Purpura
c) Raynaud's phenomenon
d) Dental caries
e) Renal tubular acidosis

33. Myasthenia gravis:

a) Is associated with thymoma
b) Never causes a sensory deficit
c) Spares the cranial nerves
d) Is accompanied by early muscle wasting
e) Is a progressive disorder

34. Which of the following cutaneous features are correctly paired with the appropriate neurocutaneous syndrome?

a) Strawberry naevus – Sturge–Weber syndrome
b) Ash leaf patch – neurofibromatosis
c) Café au lait spots – tuberous sclerosis
d) Casal's necklace – pellagra
e) Palmar pits – Gorlin's syndrome

35. Chronic subdural haematoma:

a) Results from rupture of the middle meningeal artery
b) May be associated with concealed compound fractures involving the accessory air sinuses
c) Is excluded by CT scanning
d) Usually presents with headache and lethargy
e) Is common in alcoholics

36. Down's syndrome is characterised by:

a) Autosomal recessive inheritance
b) Ostium secundum atrial septal defect
c) Prognathism
d) Trisomy 12
e) High maternal age

37. In essential hypertension:

   a) A disorder due to a single dominant gene is the probable aetiology
   b) Observer digit preference reduces measurement error in clinical trials
   c) The treatment of mild hypertension (diastolic 90–105 mmHg) is always justified
   d) An intravenous urogram is a mandatory investigation
   e) The pathognomonic pathological lesion is atheroma

38. Which of the following may cause acute polyarthritis in children?

   a) Rickets
   b) Thalassaemia
   c) Henoch–Schönlein purpura
   d) Cytomegalovirus infection
   e) Mumps

39. In coccidioidomycosis:

   a) Skin involvement is uncommon
   b) Chest pain is a common presenting feature
   c) Ketoconazole may be an effective treatment
   d) Mandibular involvement is common
   e) Sulphur granules may be seen in discharging lesions

40. Stridor may occur in:

   a) Angioedema
   b) Croup
   c) Infectious mononucleosis
   d) Bronchiectasis
   e) Systemic lupus erythematosus

41. Which of the following may be associated with a raised serum amylase?

   a) Anterior gastric ulcer
   b) Heroin injection
   c) Mesenteric infarction
   d) Syphilis
   e) Diabetic ketoacidosis

42. Predominant water depletion:

    a) Causes thirst
    b) Occurs in Addison's disease
    c) Results in secondary aldosteronism
    d) Causes hyponatraemia
    e) Complicates extensive burns

43. Causes of hypokalaemia include:

    a) Acute onset diabetes mellitus
    b) Carbenicillin therapy
    c) Renal tubular acidosis
    d) Cushing's syndrome
    e) Vitamin B_{12} therapy

44. In schizophrenia:

    a) There is inappropriate affect
    b) The CT scan is diagnostic
    c) There is anosmia
    d) There is a strong genetic tendency
    e) Auditory hallucinations are common

45. Which of the following are rare in anxiety states?

    a) Sweating
    b) Chest pain
    c) Dyspnoea
    d) Dysphagia
    e) Paraesthesia

46. Which of the following are features of Bartter's syndrome?

    a) Hyperkalaemia
    b) Gigantism
    c) Juxtaglomerular apparatus hyperplasia
    d) Increased prostaglandin E_2 excretion
    e) Women are affected more than men

47. Which of the following renal diseases are associated with multiple myeloma?

    a) Chronic renal failure
    b) Acute tubular necrosis
    c) Fanconi's syndrome
    d) Amyloidosis
    e) Nodular glomerulosclerosis

48. Renal biopsy is indicated in:

   a) Proteinuria >1 g/day with normal renal function
   b) Renal impairment in diabetics without retinopathy
   c) Polycystic kidney disease
   d) Undiagnosed chronic end-stage renal failure with small kidneys
   e) The nephrotic syndrome in adults

49. Which of the following are true of peritoneal dialysis?

   a) Creatinine clearance is higher than with haemodialysis
   b) It is contraindicated after abdominal surgery
   c) There is an increased risk of atelectasis
   d) Patients are more anaemic than with haemodialysis
   e) Patient well-being is greater than with haemodialysis

50. The adult respiratory distress syndrome may result from:

   a) Smoke inhalation
   b) Sarcoidosis
   c) Miliary tuberculosis
   d) Heroin
   e) Fat embolism

51. The diffusing capacity for carbon monoxide (DLCO) is often reduced in:

   a) Emphysema
   b) Asthma
   c) Sarcoidosis
   d) Bird fancier's lung
   e) Polycythaemia rubra vera

52. Breath sounds are increased over:

   a) Cryptogenic fibrosing alveolitis
   b) Pneumothorax
   c) The upper level of a pleural effusion
   d) Consolidation
   e) Atelectasis

53. Extrinsic allergic alveolitis may be associated with:

a) Bus conducting
b) Racing pigeons
c) Farming
d) Wine bottling
e) Cotton picking

54. Which of the following statements regarding iron absorption are true?

a) Ferrous salts are absorbed better than ferric compounds
b) Absorption is enhanced when the pH of the small bowel is low or neutral
c) Phytate-rich green vegetables increase absorption
d) Vitamin C decreases absorption
e) More than 50% of consumed iron is absorbed

55. Which of the following cells in the immune system are phagocytic?

a) Neutrophils
b) Mast cells
c) Eosinophils
d) Helper T lymphocytes
e) Alveolar macrophages

56. Familial hypertriglyceridaemia:

a) May result from lipoprotein lipase deficiency
b) Is a cause of elevated high density lipoprotein
c) Carries the greatest risk of atherogenesis of all the hyperlipidaemias
d) Is associated with tendon xanthomas
e) Is not effectively treated by diet

57. Red urine may be found with:

a) Chyluria
b) Alkaptonuria
c) Rifampicin
d) Anthrocyanin
e) Riboflavin

58. Acute hepatitis may result from:

   a) *Amanita phalloides* ingestion
   b) Pyrazinamide therapy
   c) Cytomegalovirus
   d) Wilson's disease
   e) Delta agent

59. Which of the following statements concerning statistics are true?

   a) P signifies the size of the difference between two mean values
   b) Standard deviation is twice the standard error
   c) $P < 0.1$ is taken as statistically significant
   d) Ninety per cent of observations lie within one standard deviation of the mean
   e) $Y = mc^2$ is a regression equation

60. Central cyanosis may result from:

   a) Left to right intracardiac shunt
   b) Large arteriovenous shunt in the leg
   c) Acute asthma
   d) Gastrointestinal haemorrhage
   e) Fallot's tetralogy

Examination 3

All parts of every question must be answered *True* or *False* or *Don't Know* by filling in the box provided. Failure to do so will result in rejection of the answer sheet

EXAMINATION NO.

3

SURNAME

INITIALS

Please use 2B PENCIL only. Rub out all errors thoroughly.
Mark lozenges like ▬ NOT like this ⌀ ⌀ ⌀

T ⌾ = TRUE   F ⌾ = FALSE   DK ⌾ = DON'T KNOW

	A	B	C	D	E			A	B	C	D	E
1	T F DK	T F DK	T F DK	T F DK	T F DK		16	T F DK	T F DK	T F DK	T F DK	T F DK
2	T F DK	T F DK	T F DK	T F DK	T F DK		17	T F DK	T F DK	T F DK	T F DK	T F DK
3	T F DK	T F DK	T F DK	T F DK	T F DK		18	T F DK	T F DK	T F DK	T F DK	T F DK
4	T F DK	T F DK	T F DK	T F DK	T F DK		19	T F DK	T F DK	T F DK	T F DK	T F DK
5	T F DK	T F DK	T F DK	T F DK	T F DK		20	T F DK	T F DK	T F DK	T F DK	T F DK
6	T F DK	T F DK	T F DK	T F DK	T F DK		21	T F DK	T F DK	T F DK	T F DK	T F DK
7	T F DK	T F DK	T F DK	T F DK	T F DK		22	T F DK	T F DK	T F DK	T F DK	T F DK
8	T F DK	T F DK	T F DK	T F DK	T F DK		23	T F DK	T F DK	T F DK	T F DK	T F DK
9	T F DK	T F DK	T F DK	T F DK	T F DK		24	T F DK	T F DK	T F DK	T F DK	T F DK
10	T F DK	T F DK	T F DK	T F DK	T F DK		25	T F DK	T F DK	T F DK	T F DK	T F DK
11	T F DK	T F DK	T F DK	T F DK	T F DK		26	T F DK	T F DK	T F DK	T F DK	T F DK
12	T F DK	T F DK	T F DK	T F DK	T F DK		27	T F DK	T F DK	T F DK	T F DK	T F DK
13	T F DK	T F DK	T F DK	T F DK	T F DK		28	T F DK	T F DK	T F DK	T F DK	T F DK
14	T F DK	T F DK	T F DK	T F DK	T F DK		29	T F DK	T F DK	T F DK	T F DK	T F DK
15	T F DK	T F DK	T F DK	T F DK	T F DK		30	T F DK	T F DK	T F DK	T F DK	T F DK

	A	B	C	D	E		A	B	C	D	E
31	T ☐ F ☐ DK ☐	T ☐ F ☐ DK ☐	T ☐ F ☐ DK ☐	T ☐ F ☐ DK ☐	T ☐ F ☐ DK ☐	46	T ☐ F ☐ DK ☐	T ☐ F ☐ DK ☐	T ☐ F ☐ DK ☐	T ☐ F ☐ DK ☐	T ☐ F ☐ DK ☐
32	T ☐ F ☐ DK ☐	T ☐ F ☐ DK ☐	T ☐ F ☐ DK ☐	T ☐ F ☐ DK ☐	T ☐ F ☐ DK ☐	47	T ☐ F ☐ DK ☐	T ☐ F ☐ DK ☐	T ☐ F ☐ DK ☐	T ☐ F ☐ DK ☐	T ☐ F ☐ DK ☐
33	T ☐ F ☐ DK ☐	T ☐ F ☐ DK ☐	T ☐ F ☐ DK ☐	T ☐ F ☐ DK ☐	T ☐ F ☐ DK ☐	48	T ☐ F ☐ DK ☐	T ☐ F ☐ DK ☐	T ☐ F ☐ DK ☐	T ☐ F ☐ DK ☐	T ☐ F ☐ DK ☐
34	T ☐ F ☐ DK ☐	T ☐ F ☐ DK ☐	T ☐ F ☐ DK ☐	T ☐ F ☐ DK ☐	T ☐ F ☐ DK ☐	49	T ☐ F ☐ DK ☐	T ☐ F ☐ DK ☐	T ☐ F ☐ DK ☐	T ☐ F ☐ DK ☐	T ☐ F ☐ DK ☐
35	T ☐ F ☐ DK ☐	T ☐ F ☐ DK ☐	T ☐ F ☐ DK ☐	T ☐ F ☐ DK ☐	T ☐ F ☐ DK ☐	50	T ☐ F ☐ DK ☐	T ☐ F ☐ DK ☐	T ☐ F ☐ DK ☐	T ☐ F ☐ DK ☐	T ☐ F ☐ DK ☐
36	T ☐ F ☐ DK ☐	T ☐ F ☐ DK ☐	T ☐ F ☐ DK ☐	T ☐ F ☐ DK ☐	T ☐ F ☐ DK ☐	51	T ☐ F ☐ DK ☐	T ☐ F ☐ DK ☐	T ☐ F ☐ DK ☐	T ☐ F ☐ DK ☐	T ☐ F ☐ DK ☐
37	T ☐ F ☐ DK ☐	T ☐ F ☐ DK ☐	T ☐ F ☐ DK ☐	T ☐ F ☐ DK ☐	T ☐ F ☐ DK ☐	52	T ☐ F ☐ DK ☐	T ☐ F ☐ DK ☐	T ☐ F ☐ DK ☐	T ☐ F ☐ DK ☐	T ☐ F ☐ DK ☐
38	T ☐ F ☐ DK ☐	T ☐ F ☐ DK ☐	T ☐ F ☐ DK ☐	T ☐ F ☐ DK ☐	T ☐ F ☐ DK ☐	53	T ☐ F ☐ DK ☐	T ☐ F ☐ DK ☐	T ☐ F ☐ DK ☐	T ☐ F ☐ DK ☐	T ☐ F ☐ DK ☐
39	T ☐ F ☐ DK ☐	T ☐ F ☐ DK ☐	T ☐ F ☐ DK ☐	T ☐ F ☐ DK ☐	T ☐ F ☐ DK ☐	54	T ☐ F ☐ DK ☐	T ☐ F ☐ DK ☐	T ☐ F ☐ DK ☐	T ☐ F ☐ DK ☐	T ☐ F ☐ DK ☐
40	T ☐ F ☐ DK ☐	T ☐ F ☐ DK ☐	T ☐ F ☐ DK ☐	T ☐ F ☐ DK ☐	T ☐ F ☐ DK ☐	55	T ☐ F ☐ DK ☐	T ☐ F ☐ DK ☐	T ☐ F ☐ DK ☐	T ☐ F ☐ DK ☐	T ☐ F ☐ DK ☐
41	T ☐ F ☐ DK ☐	T ☐ F ☐ DK ☐	T ☐ F ☐ DK ☐	T ☐ F ☐ DK ☐	T ☐ F ☐ DK ☐	56	T ☐ F ☐ DK ☐	T ☐ F ☐ DK ☐	T ☐ F ☐ DK ☐	T ☐ F ☐ DK ☐	T ☐ F ☐ DK ☐
42	T ☐ F ☐ DK ☐	T ☐ F ☐ DK ☐	T ☐ F ☐ DK ☐	T ☐ F ☐ DK ☐	T ☐ F ☐ DK ☐	57	T ☐ F ☐ DK ☐	T ☐ F ☐ DK ☐	T ☐ F ☐ DK ☐	T ☐ F ☐ DK ☐	T ☐ F ☐ DK ☐
43	T ☐ F ☐ DK ☐	T ☐ F ☐ DK ☐	T ☐ F ☐ DK ☐	T ☐ F ☐ DK ☐	T ☐ F ☐ DK ☐	58	T ☐ F ☐ DK ☐	T ☐ F ☐ DK ☐	T ☐ F ☐ DK ☐	T ☐ F ☐ DK ☐	T ☐ F ☐ DK ☐
44	T ☐ F ☐ DK ☐	T ☐ F ☐ DK ☐	T ☐ F ☐ DK ☐	T ☐ F ☐ DK ☐	T ☐ F ☐ DK ☐	59	T ☐ F ☐ DK ☐	T ☐ F ☐ DK ☐	T ☐ F ☐ DK ☐	T ☐ F ☐ DK ☐	T ☐ F ☐ DK ☐
45	T ☐ F ☐ DK ☐	T ☐ F ☐ DK ☐	T ☐ F ☐ DK ☐	T ☐ F ☐ DK ☐	T ☐ F ☐ DK ☐	60	T ☐ F ☐ DK ☐	T ☐ F ☐ DK ☐	T ☐ F ☐ DK ☐	T ☐ F ☐ DK ☐	T ☐ F ☐ DK ☐

1. Which of the following drugs undergo substantial first-pass metabolism?

   a) Dextropropoxyphene
   b) Propranolol
   c) Digoxin
   d) Glyceryl trinitrate
   e) Amitriptyline

2. Concerning receptors:

   a) Alpha-2 adrenoreceptors are found predominantly in vascular smooth muscle
   b) Metoclopramide is a dopaminergic antagonist
   c) Tricyclic drugs are nicotine cholinoceptor antagonists
   d) Baclofen is an antagonist of γ-aminobutyric acid
   e) Tardive dyskinesia may be related to down-regulation of dopamine receptors during the chronic administration of neuroleptics

3. In the management of cardiovascular disease:

   a) Verapamil and a beta blocker is a useful combination in heart failure
   b) Class 3 antiarrhythmics predominantly alter the rate of rise of the cardiac action potential
   c) Verapamil may precipitate digoxin toxicity
   d) Angiotensin converting enzyme inhibitors are largely excreted unchanged by the kidney
   e) Hydralazine-induced lupus occurs in approximately 5% of fast acetylators

4. Regarding the use of topical corticosteroids:

   a) Fluorination of the molecule increases the potency
   b) Clobetasone butyrate is more potent than clobetasol propionate
   c) Tinea incognito may be a side-effect
   d) They may inhibit dermal collagen synthesis
   e) They are the treatment of choice for rosacea

5. Neurological side-effects of the oral contraceptive pill include:

   a) Cerebrovascular accident
   b) Chorea
   c) Epilepsy
   d) Benign intracranial hypertension
   e) Migraine

6. Heroin:

   a) Withdrawal may be associated with rhinorrhoea and excessive lachrymation
   b) Abuse is associated with focal glomerular sclerosis
   c) May be prescribed to addicts by any post-registration physician
   d) Is not absorbed from the gastrointestinal tract
   e) Abuse by the intravenous route may be associated with fungal endocarditis

7. Which of the following indicate chronic rather than acute renal failure?

   a) Oliguria
   b) Anaemia
   c) Hypertension
   d) Bilateral small kidneys
   e) Hyperphosphataemia

8. Which of the following are causes of secondary hyperlipidaemia?

   a) Thyrotoxicosis
   b) Psoriasis
   c) Diabetes
   d) Cholestatic jaundice
   e) Retinoids

9. Recurrent hypoglycaemia is more common in diabetics with:

   a) Adrenal insufficiency
   b) Coeliac disease
   c) Autonomic neuropathy
   d) Insulinoma
   e) Long-term disease

10. Hyperkalaemia can cause which of the following ECG changes?

    a) Tall U wave
    b) Absent T wave
    c) Short QT interval
    d) Peaked P waves
    e) Narrow QRS complexes

11. Hypercalcaemia may result from:

    a) Steroid therapy
    b) Sarcoidosis
    c) Hypoparathyroidism
    d) Squamous cell carcinoma of the bronchus
    e) Multiple myeloma

12. The incubation period of which of the following diseases is less than 1 week?

    a) Filariasis
    b) Syphilis
    c) Amoebiasis
    d) Gonorrhoea
    e) Hepatitis A

13. Which of the following are mediated by exotoxins?

    a) Gram-negative sepsis
    b) Tetanus
    c) Botulism
    d) Legionnaire's disease
    e) Sleeping sickness

14. Features of lead poisoning include:

    a) Haemolytic anaemia with basophilic stippling
    b) Colicky abdominal pain
    c) Premature loss of teeth
    d) Hyperuricaemia
    e) Increased coproporphyrin III

15. Causes of anosmia include:

    a) Cushing's disease
    b) Kallmann's syndrome
    c) Tabes dorsalis
    d) Head injury
    e) Cerebral anoxia

16. Reduced urinary excretion of uric acid may be observed in which of these situations?

    a) Chronic renal disease
    b) Lesch–Nyhan syndrome
    c) Myeloma
    d) Down's syndrome
    e) Low-dose aspirin

17. Which of the following are features of pseudohypoparathyroidism?

    a) Short fourth and fifth metacarpals
    b) Hypocalcaemia
    c) Hypercalciuria
    d) Clavicular erosions
    e) Intracerebral calcification

18. Which of the following are radiological signs of hyperparathyroidism?

    a) Nephrocalcinosis
    b) Chondrocalcinosis
    c) Apical pulmonary calcification
    d) Clavicular erosions
    e) Intracerebral calcification

19. Which of the following require conversion to their active metabolite?

    a) Cyclophosphamide
    b) Rifampicin
    c) Paracetamol
    d) Prednisone
    e) Allopurinol

20. The complications of parenteral nutrition may include:

    a) Lactic acidosis
    b) Fatty liver
    c) Oesophageal stricture
    d) Osteomalacia
    e) Dermatitis

21. Which of the following are found in Marfan's syndrome?

    a) Iridodonesis
    b) Autosomal dominant inheritance
    c) Increased type 1 and decreased type 2 collagen
    d) Joint hypermobility
    e) Arm span greater than height

22. Hypertension may cause:

    a) Subdural haematoma
    b) Encephalopathy
    c) Lacunar infarcts
    d) Intracranial haemorrhage
    e) Phakoma

23. Ciliary dysfunction may lead to:

    a) Dextrocardia
    b) Mitral stenosis
    c) Infertility
    d) Recurrent pneumonia
    e) Argyll Robertson pupil

24. Pulmonary fibrosis typically causes which of the following?

    a) Increased static compliance
    b) Reduced forced expiratory volume in 1 second
    c) Enlarged right ventricle on examination
    d) Decreased alveolar–arterial oxygen gradient
    e) Increased lymphocyte count in bronchoalveolar lavage

25. Which of the following are often found in asthma?

    a) Decreased static compliance
    b) Abnormal ventilation–perfusion ratio on radioisotope lung scan
    c) Increased mast cells in bronchoalveolar lavage
    d) Increased ratio of forced expiratory volume in 1 second to forced vital capacity
    e) Very low gas transfer (DLCO)

26. Which of the following are features of alpha-1 antitrypsin deficiency?

    a) Apical hyperlucency on chest X-ray in young adults
    b) Basal bronchiectasis
    c) Dextrocardia
    d) Infertility
    e) Angiosarcoma of the liver

27. Which of the following diseases are correctly linked with their insect vector?

    a) Onchocerciasis – sand flies
    b) Falciparum malaria – *Aedes aegypti*
    c) Guinea worm disease – *Chrysops*
    d) African trypanosomiasis – Simulian black fly
    e) Chagas' disease – *Pediculus humanus corporis*

28. Hyperbaric oxygen therapy is indicated for which of the following?

    a) Crohn's disease
    b) Guillain–Barré syndrome
    c) Caisson disease
    d) Air embolism
    e) Gas gangrene

29. Which of the following are causes of pulmonary granulomata?

    a) Levi Strauss syndrome
    b) Berylliosis
    c) Sarcoidosis
    d) Histoplasmosis
    e) Chickenpox pneumonia

30. Which of the following support a diagnosis of Bechçet's syndrome?

a) Painless genital ulcers
b) HLA B27
c) Female gender
d) Sacroileitis
e) Conjunctivitis

31. Charcot's joints may result from:

a) Diabetes mellitus
b) Paget's disease
c) Rheumatoid arthritis
d) Leprosy
e) Syphilis

32. Which of the following agents may improve the clinical course of infection with the corresponding virus?

a) Pooled gamma globulin – hepatitis B
b) Acyclovir – varicella zoster
c) Amantadine – influenza A virus
d) Azathymidine – HIV
e) Prednisolone – Epstein–Barr virus

33. Cigarette smoking has been implicated in the causation of which of the following cancers?

a) Bladder
b) Bronchus
c) Cervix
d) Oesophagus
e) Thyroid

34. A soft first heart sound is found with:

a) Mitral regurgitation
b) Sinus tachycardia
c) Wolff–Parkinson–White syndrome
d) Pericardial effusion
e) Emphysema

35. Which of the following are features of atopic eczema?

a) Spongiosis
b) Elevated IgE
c) Abnormal cell-mediated immunity
d) Increased incidence of neoplastic skin disease
e) Predisposition to systemic infections

36. A stiff neck in a child of 6 months may result from:

a) Henoch–Schönlein purpura
b) Acute lymphoblastic leukaemia
c) Meningococcal meningitis
d) Lead poisoning
e) Lobar pneumonia

37. Which of the following are common in depression?

a) Structural lesions in the limbic system
b) Appetite loss
c) Insomnia
d) Constipation
e) Dementia

38. Which of the following statements about statistics are true:

a) r values are derived from t tests
b) There are usually $n+1$ degrees of freedom
c) To use a chi-square test the normal distribution needs logarithmic transformation
d) Fisher's exact test is used for small numbers
e) Statistical and clinical significance are synonymous

39. Which of the following support the diagnosis of rheumatic fever?

a) Pulmonary nodules
b) Erythema induratum
c) Huntington's chorea
d) Polyarthritis
e) Prolonged PR interval

40. Which of the following are recognised causes of thrombocytosis?

a) Splenectomy
b) von Willebrand's disease
c) Uraemia
d) Rheumatoid arthritis
e) Acute haemorrhage

41. Malabsorption may result from:

a) Primary biliary cirrhosis
b) Ulcerative colitis
c) Scleroderma
d) Hypervitaminosis A
e) Whipple's disease

42. Large pupils may be found in:

a) Horner's syndrome
b) Amphetamine addiction
c) Argyll Robertson pupil
d) Holmes–Adie pupil
e) Heroin addiction

43. Transudative ascites may result from:

a) Tuberculosis
b) Myxoedema
c) Meigs' syndrome
d) Budd–Chiari syndrome
e) Pancreatitis

44. Which of the following cause a secretory diarrhoea?

a) Prostaglandins
b) Magnesium salts
c) Cholera toxin
d) Calcitonin
e) Coeliac disease

45. Right bundle branch block is observed in:

a) Atrial septal defect
b) Pulmonary embolus
c) Pericarditis
d) Dissecting aneurysm
e) Acute pancreatitis

46. Which of the following vaccinations are routinely offered in infancy:

a) Poliomyelitis
b) BCG
c) Rubella
d) Vaccinia
e) Hepatitis B

47. Petit mal epilepsy:

a) Is associated with lesions in the parahippocampal area
b) Rarely continues into adulthood
c) Produces generalised seizures in about one-third of affected children
d) Has seizures which may be brought on by hyperventilation
e) Is associated with mental retardation

48. Causes of hypothyroidism include:

a) Sarcoidosis
b) Medullary carcinoma of the thyroid
c) Amiodarone
d) Neurofibromatosis
e) Hashimoto's disease

49. Regarding the pathophysiology of essential hypertension:

a) Angiotensin II decreases aldosterone production
b) Inhibition of slow-channel calcium entry into vascular smooth muscle leads to its relaxation
c) Renin levels may be low
d) The crucial β-adrenoceptors are in the kidney
e) End-organ capillary autonomic innervation is deranged

50. Blood transfusion may be complicated by:

a) Brucellosis
b) Post-transfusion purpura
c) Graft-versus-host disease
d) Urticaria
e) Chagas' disease

51. Erythropoietin:
    a) Deficiency is the most important cause of the anaemia of chronic renal failure
    b) Is a steroid hormone
    c) Reverses the anaemia in patients on haemodialysis
    d) Is obtained by gene cloning and expression in *E. coli*
    e) Treatment may be complicated by labile hypertension

52. γ-Interferon:
    a) Principally activates lymphocytes
    b) Tends to enhance leukotriene production in its target cells
    c) Is most effective in hairy cell leukaemia and chronic granulocytic leukaemia
    d) Has more severe side-effects than α-interferon
    e) Is a lymphokine

53. Concerning vertebral subluxation in rheumatoid arthritis:
    a) It is more likely in long-standing disease
    b) It is less frequent amongst those treated with steroids
    c) Atlanto-axial subluxation is more serious than subaxial subluxation
    d) Subaxial subluxation usually occurs at the level of C5 or C6
    e) Pain radiating from the occiput to the forehead is the classical symptom of atlanto-axial subluxation

54. Which of the following nerves and muscles are correctly paired?
    a) Pelvic nerves (nervi erigentes) – internal sphincter of the bladder
    b) Pudendal nerves – external sphincter of the bladder
    c) Glossopharyngeal nerve – cricopharyngeus
    d) Ulnar nerve – interossei
    e) Superior laryngeal nerve – intrinsic laryngeal muscles

55. Absent knee and ankle jerks with extensor plantars occur in:

a) Friedreich's ataxia
b) Multiple sclerosis
c) Subacute combined degeneration of the cord
d) L3–L4 disc protrusion
e) Myelopathy secondary to cervical spondylosis

56. Calcitonin:

a) Is a single chain polypeptide
b) Inhibits bone resorption
c) Is produced by medullary cell carcinoma
d) Inhibits urinary phosphate reabsorption
e) Is of certain benefit in osteogenesis imperfecta

57. *Chlamydia trachomatis* may cause:

a) Granuloma inguinale
b) Lymphogranuloma venereum
c) Neonatal conjunctivitis
d) Nonspecific urethritis
e) Reiter's syndrome

58. Psittacosis is:

a) Caused by a virus
b) Best treated with ampicillin
c) Associated with headache
d) Commonly transmitted man to man
e) Only definitively diagnosed on serological testing

59. Therapeutic radiation to the mediastinum causes:

a) Myasthenia gravis
b) Acute oesophagitis
c) T wave changes on ECG
d) Basal cell carcinoma
e) Prolonged PT time

60. Which of the following are side-effects of salbutamol?

a) Hyperkalaemia
b) Hyperglycaemia
c) Tremor
d) Raynaud's phenomenon
e) Hyperprolactinaemia

Examination 4

	A	B	C	D	E			A	B	C	D	E
1	T F DK	T F DK	T F DK	T F DK	T F DK		**16**	T F DK	T F DK	T F DK	T F DK	T F DK
2	T F DK	T F DK	T F DK	T F DK	T F DK		**17**	T F DK	T F DK	T F DK	T F DK	T F DK
3	T F DK	T F DK	T F DK	T F DK	T F DK		**18**	T F DK	T F DK	T F DK	T F DK	T F DK
4	T F DK	T F DK	T F DK	T F DK	T F DK		**19**	T F DK	T F DK	T F DK	T F DK	T F DK
5	T F DK	T F DK	T F DK	T F DK	T F DK		**20**	T F DK	T F DK	T F DK	T F DK	T F DK
6	T F DK	T F DK	T F DK	T F DK	T F DK		**21**	T F DK	T F DK	T F DK	T F DK	T F DK
7	T F DK	T F DK	T F DK	T F DK	T F DK		**22**	T F DK	T F DK	T F DK	T F DK	T F DK
8	T F DK	T F DK	T F DK	T F DK	T F DK		**23**	T F DK	T F DK	T F DK	T F DK	T F DK
9	T F DK	T F DK	T F DK	T F DK	T F DK		**24**	T F DK	T F DK	T F DK	T F DK	T F DK
10	T F DK	T F DK	T F DK	T F DK	T F DK		**25**	T F DK	T F DK	T F DK	T F DK	T F DK
11	T F DK	T F DK	T F DK	T F DK	T F DK		**26**	T F DK	T F DK	T F DK	T F DK	T F DK
12	T F DK	T F DK	T F DK	T F DK	T F DK		**27**	T F DK	T F DK	T F DK	T F DK	T F DK
13	T F DK	T F DK	T F DK	T F DK	T F DK		**28**	T F DK	T F DK	T F DK	T F DK	T F DK
14	T F DK	T F DK	T F DK	T F DK	T F DK		**29**	T F DK	T F DK	T F DK	T F DK	T F DK
15	T F DK	T F DK	T F DK	T F DK	T F DK		**30**	T F DK	T F DK	T F DK	T F DK	T F DK

	A	B	C	D	E		A	B	C	D	E
31	T / F / DK	T / F / DK	T / F / DK	T / F / DK	T / F / DK	46	T / F / DK	T / F / DK	T / F / DK	T / F / DK	T / F / DK
32	T / F / DK	T / F / DK	T / F / DK	T / F / DK	T / F / DK	47	T / F / DK	T / F / DK	T / F / DK	T / F / DK	T / F / DK
33	T / F / DK	T / F / DK	T / F / DK	T / F / DK	T / F / DK	48	T / F / DK	T / F / DK	T / F / DK	T / F / DK	T / F / DK
34	T / F / DK	T / F / DK	T / F / DK	T / F / DK	T / F / DK	49	T / F / DK	T / F / DK	T / F / DK	T / F / DK	T / F / DK
35	T / F / DK	T / F / DK	T / F / DK	T / F / DK	T / F / DK	50	T / F / DK	T / F / DK	T / F / DK	T / F / DK	T / F / DK
36	T / F / DK	T / F / DK	T / F / DK	T / F / DK	T / F / DK	51	T / F / DK	T / F / DK	T / F / DK	T / F / DK	T / F / DK
37	T / F / DK	T / F / DK	T / F / DK	T / F / DK	T / F / DK	52	T / F / DK	T / F / DK	T / F / DK	T / F / DK	T / F / DK
38	T / F / DK	T / F / DK	T / F / DK	T / F / DK	T / F / DK	53	T / F / DK	T / F / DK	T / F / DK	T / F / DK	T / F / DK
39	T / F / DK	T / F / DK	T / F / DK	T / F / DK	T / F / DK	54	T / F / DK	T / F / DK	T / F / DK	T / F / DK	T / F / DK
40	T / F / DK	T / F / DK	T / F / DK	T / F / DK	T / F / DK	55	T / F / DK	T / F / DK	T / F / DK	T / F / DK	T / F / DK
41	T / F / DK	T / F / DK	T / F / DK	T / F / DK	T / F / DK	56	T / F / DK	T / F / DK	T / F / DK	T / F / DK	T / F / DK
42	T / F / DK	T / F / DK	T / F / DK	T / F / DK	T / F / DK	57	T / F / DK	T / F / DK	T / F / DK	T / F / DK	T / F / DK
43	T / F / DK	T / F / DK	T / F / DK	T / F / DK	T / F / DK	58	T / F / DK	T / F / DK	T / F / DK	T / F / DK	T / F / DK
44	T / F / DK	T / F / DK	T / F / DK	T / F / DK	T / F / DK	59	T / F / DK	T / F / DK	T / F / DK	T / F / DK	T / F / DK
45	T / F / DK	T / F / DK	T / F / DK	T / F / DK	T / F / DK	60	T / F / DK	T / F / DK	T / F / DK	T / F / DK	T / F / DK

1. Pulmonary complications of rheumatoid arthritis may include:

   a) Pleural effusions
   b) Bronchiectasis
   c) Fibrosis
   d) Nodules
   e) Stridor

2. The differential diagnosis of sacroileitis includes:

   a) Gout
   b) Familial Mediterranean fever
   c) Psoriasis
   d) Reiter's syndrome
   e) Behçet's syndrome

3. Which of the following are aetiological factors in colorectal cancer?

   a) Villous adenoma
   b) Gardner's syndrome
   c) Amoebiasis
   d) Crohn's disease
   e) Multiple polyposis

4. Paradoxical splitting of the second heart sound is found in:

   a) Atrial septal defect
   b) Right ventricular failure
   c) Patent ductus arteriosus
   d) Left bundle branch block
   e) Severe aortic incompetence

5. In mitral stenosis, which of the following indicate severity?

   a) First heart sound
   b) Presystolic accentuation
   c) Late opening snap
   d) Loud opening snap
   e) Inaudible murmur

6. Mercury poisoning may be recognised by:

   a) Sunflower cataracts
   b) Demyelination
   c) Irregular tremor (Hatter's shakes)
   d) Concentric visual field loss
   e) Erethism

7. Clinical features of frontal lobe lesions include:

   a) Astereognosis
   b) Receptive dysphasia
   c) Homonymous hemianopia
   d) Muscle wasting
   e) Auditory hallucinations

8. Clinical features of the sleep apnoea syndrome include:

   a) Daytime hyperactivity
   b) Enuresis
   c) Impotence
   d) Snoring
   e) Angina pectoris

9. Which of the following tests elucidate disease of the large airways?

   a) Closing volumes
   b) Static compliance
   c) Gas transfer
   d) Flow volume curves at low lung volumes
   e) Peak flow

10. Which of the following statements are true:

   a) Depression complicating hypothyroidism in the elderly may require electroconvulsive therapy
   b) Mania increases in incidence with age
   c) Senile dementia due to vascular disease is more common than the Alzheimer type
   d) Part II accommodation refers to a section of the National Assistance Act (1948)
   e) Multi-infarct dementia may be complicated by fits

11. Hyperchloraemic acidosis (normal anion gap) may result from:

   a) Uraemia
   b) Renal tubular acidosis
   c) Diabetes mellitus
   d) Acetazolamide
   e) Diarrhoea in neonates

12. Hypophosphataemia:

   a) May result from distal renal tubular dysfunction
   b) Is associated with polycythaemia
   c) May complicate parenteral nutrition
   d) Occurs during the treatment of diabetic ketoacidosis
   e) May cause rhabdomyolysis

13. Methotrexate may cause:

   a) Malabsorption
   b) Photosensitivity
   c) Pneumonitis
   d) Haemorrhagic cystitis
   e) Conjunctivitis

14. The phrenic nerve:

   a) Is derived mainly from C6
   b) Is the sole motor nerve to the diaphragm
   c) Is sensory to the diaphragmatic pleura
   d) Is functioning normally if downward movement of the diaphragm occurs on sniffing during fluoroscopy
   e) Is sensory to the pericardium

15. Haemoglobinuria occurs with:

   a) Acute glomerulonephritis
   b) Henoch–Schönlein purpura
   c) *Clostridium welchii* septicaemia
   d) Methaemoglobinaemia
   e) Marathon running

16. The third heart sound:

    a) Is abnormal in healthy people
    b) Is a sign of constrictive pericarditis
    c) Occurs when Eisenmenger's syndrome complicates a
       ventricular septal defect
    d) Occurs in mitral stenosis
    e) Occurs 0.5 seconds after the second sound

17. Peritonitis complicating chronic ambulatory peritoneal
    dialysis:

    a) Is commonly caused by fungi
    b) Is usually due to intestinal microorganisms
    c) Is best prevented by long-term prophylactic antibiotic
       administration
    d) Is frequently accompanied by clinical symptoms and
       signs
    e) Is the commonest complication

18. Causes of hair loss include:

    a) Systemic lupus erythematosus
    b) Minoxidil
    c) Chloroambucil
    d) Retinoids
    e) Lichen planus

19. Which of the following root values are correct?

    a) Deltoid/C3–C4
    b) Finger flexors/C4–C5
    c) Triceps/C5
    d) Radial nerve/C7–T1
    e) Median nerve/C5–C7

20. A central scotoma occurs with:

    a) Retrobulbar neuritis
    b) Senile macular degeneration
    c) Tobacco amblyopia
    d) Glaucoma
    e) Retinitis pigmentosa

21. Acute epiglottitis:

   a) Is usually caused by *H. influenzae* type b
   b) Is associated with salivary drooling
   c) Is associated with septicaemia
   d) Is best diagnosed by a throat swab
   e) Is a disease of 4–10-year-olds

22. Causes of anaemia with splenomegaly in a child include:

   a) Thalassaemia
   b) Congenital spherocytosis
   c) Gaucher's disease
   d) Portal vein thrombosis
   e) Idiopathic thrombocytopenic purpura

23. Measles encephalitis:

   a) Has an onset within a week of the rash appearing
   b) Is excluded by a normal lumbar puncture
   c) Is effectively treated with acyclovir
   d) Commonly progresses to subacute sclerosing panencephalitis
   e) Is indicated by a seizure during the febrile stage

24. Cutaneous manifestations of TB include:

   a) Erythema nodosum
   b) Erythema marginatum
   c) Lupus vulgaris
   d) Pyoderma gangrenosum
   e) Phlyctenular conjunctivitis

25. Acquired circulating inhibitors of coagulation:

   a) Are normally IgM heavy chains
   b) Occur in 70% of haemophiliacs
   c) Cause serious gastrointestinal haemorrhage
   d) Are associated with penicillin hypersensitivity reactions
   e) Are associated with recurrent abortions

26. IgE:

   a) Is synthesised by mast cells
   b) Is composed of two heavy and two light chains
   c) Is found in the highest concentrations in patients with atopic eczema
   d) Has a mean serum concentration of 0.5 g/l
   e) Is implicated in the Prausnitz–Küstner reaction

27. Classical features of schizophrenia are:

   a) Visual hallucinations
   b) Incongruity of mood
   c) Feelings of passivity
   d) Paranoid delusions
   e) Thought insertion

28. Mania:

   a) Occurs in cyclothymic personalities
   b) May progress to hypermania
   c) May lead to promiscuity
   d) May be treated with carbamazepine
   e) Presents with auditory hallucinations

29. Contraindications for pertussis vaccine may include:

   a) Down's syndrome
   b) Cystic fibrosis
   c) Congenital heart disease
   d) Benign febrile convulsions in a sibling
   e) Petit mal in a sibling

30. Pericardial tamponade:

   a) May be due to aortic dissection
   b) Is suggested by a brachial pulse that disappears on inspiration
   c) Is best treated by diuretics
   d) Causes the jugular venous pressure to rise on inspiration
   e) Is differentiated from congestive cardiac failure by the absence of hepatomegaly

31. Which of the following drugs may precipitate digoxin toxicity in the elderly?

a) Kaolin/morphine
b) Quinine sulphate
c) Erythromycin
d) Metoclopramide
e) Diuretics

32. In ostium secundum atrial septal defect:

a) Atrial fibrillation may occur
b) Spontaneous closure occurs in 10% of cases
c) Subacute bacterial endocarditis is commoner than in a ventricular septal defect
d) The onset of pulmonary hypertension is usually in childhood
e) Eisenmenger's syndrome is an indication for surgery

33. Mast cells are involved in:

a) Cold urticaria
b) Urticaria after strawberry consumption
c) Tuberculin anaphylaxis
d) Bee sting reaction
e) Serum sickness

34. Causes of lumps in the mouth include:

a) Palatal tori
b) Kaposi's sarcoma
c) Behçet's syndrome
d) Pyogenic granuloma
e) Fordyce's spots

35. Which of the following discolour the urine?

a) Beetroot
b) Tetracyclines
c) Methyldopa
d) Rifampicin
e) Homogentisic acid

36. Patients with a pituitary adenoma may have:

   a) Hypertension
   b) Loss of body hair
   c) Impotence
   d) Glycosuria
   e) Hyperprolactinaemia

37. Which of the following are causes of short stature?

   a) Turner's syndrome
   b) Klinefelter's syndrome
   c) Down's syndrome
   d) Crohn's disease
   e) Atopic eczema

38. Tissue-specific antibodies are aetiologically important in:

   a) Primary hyperaldosteronism
   b) Ulcerative colitis
   c) Pernicious anaemia
   d) Myasthenia gravis
   e) Thyrotoxicosis with exophthalmos

39. Which of the following names and diseases are correctly associated?

   a) Rachmaninov – acromegaly
   b) Robbie Burns – rheumatic fever
   c) Joan of Arc – tuberculosis
   d) John Hunter – syphilis
   e) Lewis Carroll – migraine

40. By the age of 1 year a child should be able to:

   a) Tie shoelaces
   b) Copy a circle with a pencil
   c) Turn the pages of a book
   d) Seat himself on a chair
   e) Walk supported by one hand

41. Common features of chronic subdural haematoma include:

   a) Tachycardia
   b) Pupillary signs
   c) Fluctuating level of consciousness
   d) Normal cerebrospinal fluid
   e) Neck stiffness

42. A good response to oral steroids is expected in:

   a) Childhood nephrotic syndrome
   b) Minimal change glomerulonephritis
   c) Ankylosing spondylitis
   d) Landry's paralysis
   e) Toxic epidermal necrolysis

43. Which of the following drugs produce hyponatraemia?

   a) Carbamazepine
   b) Demeclocycline
   c) Lithium
   d) Chlorpropamide
   e) Amitriptyline

44. In subphrenic abscess:

   a) The left side is more commonly affected than the right
   b) Rigors are common
   c) Pleural effusion may occur
   d) A fluid level indicates rupture into the thorax
   e) Patients may hiccough

45. Huntington's chorea:

   a) Presents at between 30 and 50 years
   b) In children may present with rigidity
   c) Responds well to penicillamine
   d) Is inherited as an autosomal dominant condition
   e) May present to a psychiatrist

46. In hypophosphatasia:

   a) Vitamin D is a satisfactory treatment
   b) The inheritance is probably recessive
   c) The serum phosphate is low
   d) Bone fractures and an elevated serum alkaline
      phosphatase are common features
   e) Increased phosphoethanolamine excretion in the urine is
      pathognomonic

47. Electroconvulsive therapy:

a) Is associated less with memory loss when both electrodes are placed over the non-dominant hemisphere
b) Is contraindicated by raised intracranial pressure
c) Is contraindicated by concomitant monoamine oxidase inhibitor treatment
d) Cannot be given without consent
e) Improves depression more swiftly than drugs

48. Carcinoma associated with ulcerative colitis:

a) Is commoner in pancolitis
b) Is more frequent if disease has been present for less than 10 years
c) May be present at multiple sites in the colon
d) May affect the bile duct
e) Commonly presents with a change in symptoms

49. Causes of generalised pruritus include:

a) Atopic eczema
b) Iron deficiency with normal full blood count and red cell indices
c) Polycythaemia rubra vera
d) Long-standing renal failure
e) Occult malignancy

50. The following influence transfer factor (DLCO):

a) Haemoglobin concentration
b) Cigarette smoking immediately before testing
c) Intrapulmonary haemorrhage
d) Uraemia
e) Lung volume at the time of measurement

51. Childhood wheezing may be due to:

a) Epiglottitis
b) Alpha-1 antitrypsin deficiency
c) Mediastinal cyst
d) Hypovitaminosis A
e) Cannabis

52. Facial palsy in the older child may be due to:

   a) Nuclear agenesis
   b) A post-ictal event
   c) Möbius' syndrome
   d) Henoch–Schönlein purpura
   e) Sarcoidosis

53. Immune complexes are implicated in which of the following diseases?

   a) Malaria
   b) Parkinson's disease
   c) Sarcoidosis
   d) Subacute bacterial endocarditis
   e) Leprosy

54. Which of the following equations are correctly phrased?

   a) MCV = PCV/MCH
   b) pH = pK + log [Base]/ [Acid]
   c) FEV_1 + ERV = RV
   d) $C = \dfrac{[U]}{[S]} \times$ Volume
   e) Standard deviation = $\sqrt{\sum \dfrac{(\text{Value} - \text{Mean})^2}{\text{Number of patients}}}$

55. Which of the following statements are true?

   a) Half of the population have an IQ of less than 150
   b) A woman with Down's syndrome may give birth to a normal infant
   c) Mental subnormality may be due to maternal toxaemia
   d) Autistic children are often over-active
   e) Giggles incontinence suggests sacral agenesis

56. Warm autoimmune haemolytic anaemia may be associated with:

   a) Donath–Landsteiner antibody
   b) *Mycoplasma* pneumonia
   c) Evans' syndrome
   d) Systemic lupus erythematosus
   e) Hydrops fetalis

57. Under which of the following circumstances may brain death be diagnosed?

   a) The diagnosis of a disorder which can lead to brain death must be established
   b) Both vestibulo-ocular reflexes must be shown to be absent
   c) The patient is being ventilated
   d) There is no evidence of hypothermia
   e) Diagnostic tests must always be repeated

58. Temporal (giant cell) arteritis may present with:

   a) A normal erythrocyte sedimentation rate
   b) Limb claudication
   c) Raynaud's phenomenon
   d) Photosensitivity
   e) Anaemia

59. Which of the following vitamins are correctly paired with their major dietary source?

   a) Vitamin A – green vegetables
   b) Vitamin B – polished rice
   c) Vitamin C – milk
   d) Vitamin D – fish
   e) Vitamin E – polar bear liver

60. An instrument or test:

   a) Is specific if there are few false negatives
   b) Is sensitive if there are many true negatives
   c) Is precise if the validity is high
   d) Has a high predictive value if the proportion of negative results that are true negatives is high
   e) Is accurate if the validity is high

Examination 5

SURNAME

INITIALS

Please use 2B PENCIL only. Rub out all errors thoroughly.
Mark lozenges like ⬤ NOT like this ∅ ∅ ⊗

T ⊂⊃ = TRUE   F ⊂⊃ = FALSE   DK ⊂⊃ = DON'T KNOW

	A	B	C	D	E			A	B	C	D	E
1	T F DK	T F DK	T F DK	T F DK	T F DK		**16**	T F DK	T F DK	T F DK	T F DK	T F DK
2	T F DK	T F DK	T F DK	T F DK	T F DK		**17**	T F DK	T F DK	T F DK	T F DK	T F DK
3	T F DK	T F DK	T F DK	T F DK	T F DK		**18**	T F DK	T F DK	T F DK	T F DK	T F DK
4	T F DK	T F DK	T F DK	T F DK	T F DK		**19**	T F DK	T F DK	T F DK	T F DK	T F DK
5	T F DK	T F DK	T F DK	T F DK	T F DK		**20**	T F DK	T F DK	T F DK	T F DK	T F DK
6	T F DK	T F DK	T F DK	T F DK	T F DK		**21**	T F DK	T F DK	T F DK	T F DK	T F DK
7	T F DK	T F DK	T F DK	T F DK	T F DK		**22**	T F DK	T F DK	T F DK	T F DK	T F DK
8	T F DK	T F DK	T F DK	T F DK	T F DK		**23**	T F DK	T F DK	T F DK	T F DK	T F DK
9	T F DK	T F DK	T F DK	T F DK	T F DK		**24**	T F DK	T F DK	T F DK	T F DK	T F DK
10	T F DK	T F DK	T F DK	T F DK	T F DK		**25**	T F DK	T F DK	T F DK	T F DK	T F DK
11	T F DK	T F DK	T F DK	T F DK	T F DK		**26**	T F DK	T F DK	T F DK	T F DK	T F DK
12	T F DK	T F DK	T F DK	T F DK	T F DK		**27**	T F DK	T F DK	T F DK	T F DK	T F DK
13	T F DK	T F DK	T F DK	T F DK	T F DK		**28**	T F DK	T F DK	T F DK	T F DK	T F DK
14	T F DK	T F DK	T F DK	T F DK	T F DK		**29**	T F DK	T F DK	T F DK	T F DK	T F DK
15	T F DK	T F DK	T F DK	T F DK	T F DK		**30**	T F DK	T F DK	T F DK	T F DK	T F DK

	A	B	C	D	E		A	B	C	D	E
31	T F DK	T F DK	T F DK	T F DK	T F DK	46	T F DK	T F DK	T F DK	T F DK	T F DK
32	T F DK	T F DK	T F DK	T F DK	T F DK	47	T F DK	T F DK	T F DK	T F DK	T F DK
33	T F DK	T F DK	T F DK	T F DK	T F DK	48	T F DK	T F DK	T F DK	T F DK	T F DK
34	T F DK	T F DK	T F DK	T F DK	T F DK	49	T F DK	T F DK	T F DK	T F DK	T F DK
35	T F DK	T F DK	T F DK	T F DK	T F DK	50	T F DK	T F DK	T F DK	T F DK	T F DK
36	T F DK	T F DK	T F DK	T F DK	T F DK	51	T F DK	T F DK	T F DK	T F DK	T F DK
37	T F DK	T F DK	T F DK	T F DK	T F DK	52	T F DK	T F DK	T F DK	T F DK	T F DK
38	T F DK	T F DK	T F DK	T F DK	T F DK	53	T F DK	T F DK	T F DK	T F DK	T F DK
39	T F DK	T F DK	T F DK	T F DK	T F DK	54	T F DK	T F DK	T F DK	T F DK	T F DK
40	T F DK	T F DK	T F DK	T F DK	T F DK	55	T F DK	T F DK	T F DK	T F DK	T F DK
41	T F DK	T F DK	T F DK	T F DK	T F DK	56	T F DK	T F DK	T F DK	T F DK	T F DK
42	T F DK	T F DK	T F DK	T F DK	T F DK	57	T F DK	T F DK	T F DK	T F DK	T F DK
43	T F DK	T F DK	T F DK	T F DK	T F DK	58	T F DK	T F DK	T F DK	T F DK	T F DK
44	T F DK	T F DK	T F DK	T F DK	T F DK	59	T F DK	T F DK	T F DK	T F DK	T F DK
45	T F DK	T F DK	T F DK	T F DK	T F DK	60	T F DK	T F DK	T F DK	T F DK	T F DK

1. Which of the following act as inhibitors of hepatic mono-oxygenase activity?

   a) Cigarette smoking
   b) Griseofulvin
   c) Cimetidine
   d) Metronidazole
   e) Co-trimoxazole

2. Which of the following drugs are definitely teratogenic in humans?

   a) Warfarin
   b) Isotretinoin
   c) Cefuroxime
   d) Methyldopa
   e) Oxytetracycline

3. Which of the following drugs are excreted largely unchanged by the kidney?

   a) Digoxin
   b) Lithium
   c) Gentamicin
   d) Aspirin
   e) Levodopa

4. Which of the following drugs may be used safely in a breast-feeding mother?

   a) Erythromycin
   b) Amiodarone
   c) Prednisolone (10 mg daily)
   d) Lithium
   e) Aspirin

5. Clinical features of hypercapnia include:

   a) Extensor plantars
   b) Fine tremor
   c) Cold peripheries
   d) Confusion
   e) Headache

6. Which of the following effects can digoxin produce on an ECG?

   a) Atrial fibrillation
   b) PR prolongation
   c) Elongation of QT
   d) ST depression
   e) Widened QRS complex

7. Right bundle branch block may be caused by:

   a) Right ventricular strain
   b) Atrial septal defect
   c) Digoxin
   d) Pulmonary embolism
   e) Normality

8. An elevated pCO_2 may be found with:

   a) Severe kyphoscoliosis
   b) Raised intracranial pressure
   c) Mild asthma
   d) Barbiturate overdoses
   e) The early stages of cryptogenic fibrosing alveolitis

9. In which of the following diseases may organisms be cultured from the bone marrow?

   a) *Pneumocystis carinii* pneumonia
   b) Typhoid
   c) Sarcoidosis
   d) Tuberculosis
   e) Brucellosis

10. Pneumococcal vaccination may be indicated for patients in which of the following categories?

   a) Newborn infants
   b) Alcoholics
   c) Elective splenectomy
   d) Lymphoma
   e) HBsAG positive

11. The incubation period of which of the following is more than 3 weeks?

    a) Herpes simplex infection
    b) Hepatitis B
    c) Visceral leishmaniasis
    d) Meningococcal meningitis
    e) Diphtheria

12. Salicylate overdosage may cause:

    a) Confabulation
    b) Hypoglycaemia
    c) Pulmonary oedema
    d) Wrist drop
    e) Sweating

13. Skin peeling is a feature of:

    a) Staphylococcal toxic shock syndrome
    b) Streptococcal infection
    c) Kawasaki disease
    d) Carcinoid syndrome
    e) Staphylococcal scalded skin syndrome

14. Bullous eruptions are features of:

    a) Pemphigoid
    b) Erythema induratum
    c) Pellagra
    d) Dermatitis herpetiformis
    e) Darier's disease

15. Ampicillin rashes are more common in which of the following conditions?

    a) Benzodiazepine therapy
    b) *Mycoplasma* pneumonia
    c) Infectious mononucleosis
    d) Chronic lymphatic leukaemia
    e) Coeliac disease

16. Lactic acidosis may result from:

    a) Metformin therapy
    b) Uraemia
    c) Cholestyramine
    d) Hypoventilation
    e) Cimetidine

17. A "rugger jersey" spine may be seen in:

    a) Paget's disease
    b) Alkaptonuria
    c) Myeloma
    d) Hodgkin's disease
    e) Renal osteodystrophy

18. Which of the following antidotes are correctly paired with a poison?

    a) Penicillamine D – thallium
    b) Desferrioxamine – Iron
    c) Amyl nitrite – cyanide
    d) Hyperbaric oxygen – carbon monoxide
    e) Sodium/calcium EDTA – lead

19. Regarding the surface markings of the thoracic contents:

    a) The trachea bifurcates just below the angle of Louis
    b) The manubrium sterni overlies the aortic arch
    c) The pleura descends below the twelfth rib posteriorly
    d) The internal mammary artery is protected by the sternum
    e) The apex of the pleura is protected by the clavicle

20. Which of the following statements are true of malaria?

    a) Prophylaxis should be continued for at least 4 weeks after leaving an endemic area
    b) *P. vivax* infection is a likely cause of fever in a West African
    c) Hypoglycaemia is a recognised complication of therapy
    d) Females may develop severe haemolysis when treated with primaquine
    e) Mosquito netting is valuable prophylaxis

21. Which of the following drugs predispose to kernicterus?

    a) Chloramphenicol
    b) Phenytoin
    c) Salbutamol
    d) Aspirin
    e) Nicotine

22. Which of the following diseases may be cured by dapsone?

    a) Leprosy
    b) Syphilis
    c) HIV infection
    d) Pyoderma gangrenosum
    e) Dermatitis herpetiformis

23. Which of the following effects occur with respect to drug metabolism in pregnancy?

    a) Increased glomerular filtration rate
    b) Increased gastric emptying
    c) Increased volume distribution
    d) Increased plasma protein binding
    e) Increased hepatic microsomal enzyme activity

24. Folate deficiency may result from which of the following?

    a) "Blind loop" syndrome
    b) Beer drinking alcoholism
    c) Digoxin
    d) Phenytoin
    e) Hereditary elliptocytosis

25. Oral contraceptives may lead to:

    a) Increased very low density lipoprotein triglycerides
    b) Bloom's disease
    c) Hepatic cirrhosis
    d) Osteoporosis
    e) Sarcoidosis

26. Which of the following suggest the possibility of a brain stem lesion?

    a) Horizontal nystagmus
    b) Internuclear ophthalmoplegia
    c) Dysphasia
    d) Opisthotonus
    e) Cerebellar signs

27. Which of the following are features of a basal pontine haemorrhage?

    a) Sweating
    b) Cheyne–Stokes respiration
    c) Lacunar infarcts
    d) Gradual onset of symptoms
    e) Good prognosis

28. Which of the following may be the cause of multiple cranial nerve palsies?

    a) Sarcoidosis
    b) Carcinomatosis
    c) Tuberculosis
    d) Paget's disease
    e) Syphilis

29. Which of the following are clinical features of intracranial arteriovenous malformations?

    a) Epilepsy
    b) Headaches
    c) Neck stiffness
    d) Strokes during pregnancy
    e) "Pepperpot" skull on X-ray

30. Clinical features of temporal lobe epilepsy include:

    a) *Jamais vu* phenomenon
    b) Micropsia
    c) Ataxia
    d) Dressing apraxia
    e) Agraphia

31. Which of the following often cause wheezing?

a) Left ventricular failure
b) Farmer's lung
c) Carcinoid tumour
d) Coal miner's pneumoconiosis
e) Asbestosis

32. Haemoptysis may result from:

a) Cryptogenic fibrosing alveolitis
b) Aspergilloma
c) Osler–Weber–Rendu syndrome
d) Bronchial adenoma
e) *Pneumocystis carinii* pneumonia

33. Basal crepitations are a clinical feature of:

a) Humidifier fever
b) Right ventricular failure
c) Emphysema
d) Post-radiation fibrosis
e) Bronchiectasis

34. Causes of bilateral hilar lymphadenopathy on chest X-ray include:

a) Infectious mononucleosis
b) Toxoplasmosis
c) Hydatid disease
d) Sarcoidosis
e) Non-Hodgkin's lymphoma

35. Multiple pulmonary nodules on chest X-ray may result from:

a) Pulmonary haemosiderosis
b) Tuberculosis
c) Histoplasmosis
d) Pneumoconiosis
e) Prostatic cancer

36. The clinical features of bronchopulmonary aspergillosis include:

a) A peripheral blood eosinophilia
b) Lower lobe fusiform bronchiectasis
c) A clinical response to inhaled amphotericin
d) A requirement for maintenance treatment with oral steroids
e) An immediate positive skin test to *Aspergillus nigricans*

37. Which of the following are causes of chylothorax?

a) Meigs' syndrome
b) Pancreatitis
c) Myxoedema
d) Lymphoma
e) Trauma

38. Physical findings in the carpal tunnel syndrome may include:

a) Hypothenar wasting
b) Weakness of opposition of the thumb
c) Loss of supinator reflex
d) Acromegaly
e) Ulnar deviation

39. Morning stiffness is characteristic of:

a) Rheumatoid arthritis
b) Osteoarthritis
c) Polymyalgia rheumatica
d) Ankylosing spondylitis
e) Reiter's syndrome

40. Tendon sheath nodules may occur in which of the following?

a) Rheumatoid arthritis
b) Gout
c) Osteoarthritis
d) Psoriasis
e) Pseudogout

41. The differential diagnosis of orogenital ulceration includes:

a) Reiter's syndrome
b) Erythema multiforme
c) Pemphigoid
d) Crohn's disease
e) Syphilis

42. Potential causes of pain in Paget's disease include:

a) Gout
b) Pseudogout
c) Pathological fractures
d) Osteoarthritis
e) Charcot's joint

43. Gout in a child may be caused by:

a) Marfan's syndrome
b) Lead poisoning
c) Sickle cell disease
d) Acute leukaemia
e) Paracetamol

44. Which of the following cancers may exhibit hormonal dependence?

a) Endometrial
b) Hypernephroma
c) Thyroid
d) Bronchial
e) Pancreatic

45. Which of the following are associated with carcinoma of the oesophagus?

a) Smoking
b) Alcohol
c) Palmar–plantar keratoderma
d) Iron deficiency
e) Vitamin B_{12} deficiency

46. When inspecting the jugular venous pulse, an absent "Y" descent is seen with:

   a) Constrictive pericarditis
   b) Tricuspid incompetence
   c) Mitral stenosis
   d) Cardiac tamponade
   e) Acute left ventricular failure

47. Features of an innocent murmur include:

   a) Diastolic timing
   b) Widespread radiation
   c) Normal ECG
   d) Single S2 in expiration
   e) Loud S1

48. The severity of mitral stenosis may be judged by:

   a) Loudness of opening snap
   b) Length of systolic murmur
   c) Timing of opening snap
   d) Presystolic accentuation
   e) The pressure across the valve at catheterisation

49. Clinical features of a left atrial myxoma may include:

   a) Normal chest X-ray
   b) Fever
   c) Loud S2
   d) Clubbing
   e) Machinery murmur

50. Mitral valve prolapse may occur in which of the following conditions?

   a) Ehlers–Danlos syndrome
   b) Marfan's syndrome
   c) Polyarteritis nodosum
   d) Ostium primum atrial septal defect
   e) Wolff–Parkinson–White syndrome

51. The features of Wilson's disease include:

    a) High serum copper
    b) Low caeruloplasmin
    c) Arcus senilis
    d) Chondrocalcinosis
    e) Diabetes mellitus

52. In a fat child who is small for his age, which of the following conditions should be considered?

    a) Hypothyroidism
    b) Hirschsprung's disease
    c) Pseudohypoparathyroidism
    d) Klinefelter's syndrome
    e) Prader–Willi syndrome

53. Photophobia in children may be due to:

    a) Wilson's disease
    b) Congenital glaucoma
    c) Maternal heroin addiction
    d) Acrodermatitis enteropathica
    e) Corneal ulcer

54. Depression in childhood may present with:

    a) Stridor
    b) Excessive eating
    c) Enuresis
    d) Abdominal pain
    e) A strong family history

55. Which of the following are causes of lymphadenopathy in children?

    a) Juvenile chronic arthritis (Still's disease)
    b) Toxoplasmosis
    c) Cystic fibrosis
    d) Caffey's disease
    e) BCG vaccination

56. In bone marrow transplantation:

   a) Bone marrow is usually obtained from the sternum
   b) Graft-versus-host disease occurs in 70% of allograft recipients
   c) Reactivation cytomegalovirus infection is a common complication
   d) All acute adult leukaemias are probably best treated in first remission
   e) Autologous grafting has the advantage that the marrow is often harvested in second or subsequent remissions

57. Kawasaki disease:

   a) Predominantly affects adults
   b) Bears a superficial resemblance to mercury intoxication
   c) Is associated with coronary artery abnormalities
   d) Responds to acyclovir
   e) Is characterised by palmar–plantar erythema with peri-ungual exfoliation

58. Cataracts are associated with:

   a) Hypothyroidism
   b) Atopic eczema
   c) Chloroquine
   d) Diabetes
   e) Infectious mononucleosis

59. In acute leukaemia:

   a) Death is usually from infection
   b) Hyperuricaemia is found at presentation
   c) Experimental treatment is often considered after the second relapse
   d) CNS prophylaxis is usually given in acute myelogenous leukaemia
   e) If the platelet count falls below 70×10^9/litre then platelet transfusion is indicated

60. Which of the following disorders are transmitted in an autosomal dominant manner?

   a) Cystic fibrosis
   b) Sickle cell anaemia
   c) Tuberous sclerosis
   d) Marfan's syndrome
   e) Acute intermittent porphyria

Answers

Examination 1

(Pass mark 160)

1. True — a, e
2. True — b, e
3. True — c, e
4. True — e
5. True — a, e
6. True — e
7. True — a, b, c, d
8. True — b, d, e
9. True — b, d
10. True — a, b, d, e
11. True — a, b, d, e
12. True — a, b, d
13. True — none
14. True — c, d
15. True — b, c, d
16. True — a, b, d, e
17. True — a, b, d
18. True — a, b, d
19. True — c, d, e
20. True — a, c, e
21. True — c, e
22. True — b, e
23. True — a, b
24. True — b, c
25. True — b, c, d
26. True — a
27. True — b
28. True — a, d, e
29. True — none
30. True — b, c, e

31. True — a, b, d
32. True — b, c, d
33. True — a, b, d
34. True — b, c, e
35. True — b, c, d, e
36. True — none
37. True — b, e
38. True — a, b, d, e
39. True — a, c
40. True — a
41. True — a, b, c, d, e
42. True — e
43. True — d, e
44. True — a, d, e
45. True — a
46. True — c
47. True — a, d
48. True — b, c, d
49. True — b, c
50. True — d, e
51. True — a, d, e
52. True — b
53. True — a, b, c, d, e
54. True — a, b, c, d
55. True — b, e
56. True — c
57. True — c, d, e
58. True — a, c, d, e
59. True — b, c
60. True — b, c, e

Examination 2

(Pass mark 165)

1. True — b, d	31. True — a, c, d, e
2. True — b, c, e	32. True — a, b, c, d, e
3. True — b, d	33. True — a, b
4. True — b, e	34. True — c, d, e
5. True — b, d, e	35. True — b, d, e
6. True — b, e	36. True — e
7. True — a, c	37. True — none
8. True — c, d, e	38. True — c, d, e
9. True — d	39. True — b, c
10. True — a, b, c, d, e	40. True — a, b, c
11. True — a, d, e	41. True — b, c, e
12. True — a, b, e	42. True — a, e
13. True — a, b, c, e	43. True — b, c, d, e
14. True — a, d, e	44. True — a, e
15. True — b, c, e	45. True — none
16. True — a, c, d	46. True — c, d, e
17. True — c, d	47. True — a, b, c, d
18. True — b, d	48. True — a, b, e
19. True — a	49. True — b, c, e
20. True — a	50. True — a, c, d, e
21. True — a, c, d, e	51. True — a, c, d
22. True — d	52. True — c, d
23. True — a, b, c, d, e	53. True — b, c
24. True — a, b, c, d, e	54. True — a, b
25. True — a, b, c, d, e	55. True — a, e
26. True — a, b, c, d, e	56. True — a, e
27. True — a, c, d, e	57. True — c, d
28. True — a, b, c	58. True — a, b, c, d, e
29. True — b, c, e	59. True — none
30. True — c, d	60. True — c, e

Examination 3

(Pass mark 160)

1. True — a, b, d, e
2. True — b
3. True — c
4. True — a, c, d
5. True — a, b, c, d, e
6. True — a, b, e
7. True — b, d, e
8. True — c, d, e
9. True — a, b, c, e
10. True — e
11. True — b, d, e
12. True — d
13. True — b, c
14. True — a, b, c, d, e
15. True — b, c, d, e
16. True — a, d, e
17. True — a, b
18. True — a, b, d
19. True — a, d
20. True — a, b, d, e
21. True — a, b, d, e
22. True — b, c, d
23. True — a, c, d
24. True — b
25. True — b, c
26. True — none
27. True — none
28. True — e
29. True — b, c, d
30. True — none

31. True — a, d, e
32. True — b, c, d, e
33. True — a, b, c, d
34. True — a, d, e
35. True — a, b, c
36. True — b, c, e
37. True — b, c, d
38. True — d
39. True — d, e
40. True — a, d, e
41. True — a, c, e
42. True — b, d
43. True — b, c, d
44. True — a, c, d
45. True — a, b
46. True — a
47. True — b, c, d
48. True — a, c, e
49. True — b, c
50. True — a, b, c, d, e
51. True — a, c, e
52. True — b, d, e
53. True — a, d, e
54. True — a, b, d
55. True — a, c
56. True — a, b, c, d
57. True — b, c, d, e
58. True — c, e
59. True — b, c, d
60. True — b, c

Examination 4

(Pass mark 135)

1. True — a, c, d
2. True — b, c, d, e
3. True — a, b, d, e
4. True — c, d, e
5. True — c
6. True — c, d, e
7. True — none
8. True — d
9. True — e
10. True — a, d, e
11. True — b, d, e
12. True — a, c, d, e
13. True — c, e
14. True — b, c, d, e
15. True — c, d, e
16. True — b
17. True — e
18. True — a, c, d, e
19. True — none
20. True — a, b, c, d
21. True — a, b, c
22. True — a, b, c
23. True — a
24. True — a, c
25. True — e
26. True — b, c, e
27. True — b, c, d, e
28. True — a, c, d
29. True — a, e
30. True — a, b, d

31. True — c, e
32. True — a
33. True — a, b, d
34. True — a, b, d, e
35. True — a, b, c, d, e
36. True — a, b, c, d, e
37. True — a, c, d, e
38. True — c, d, e
39. True — a, b, c, d, e
40. True — e
41. True — b, c
42. True — a, b
43. True — a, d, e
44. True — c, e
45. True — a, b, d, e
46. True — b, e
47. True — a, b, e
48. True — a, c, d
49. True — a, b, c, d, e
50. True — a, b, c, e
51. True — b, c, e
52. True — b, e
53. True — a, d, e
54. True — b
55. True — b, c
56. True — c, d
57. True — a, c, d,
58. True — a, b, c, e
59. True — a, d
60. True — b, d, e

Examination 5

(Pass mark 130)

1. True — c, d, e
2. True — a, b, e
3. True — a, b, c
4. True — a, c
5. True — d, e
6. True — a, b, d
7. True — a, b, d, e
8. True — a, b, d
9. True — b, d, e
10. True — b, c, d
11. True — b, c
12. True — b, c, e
13. True — b, c, e
14. True — a, d
15. True — c, d
16. True — a, b, d
17. True — e
18. True — b, c, d, e
19. True — a, b, c
20. True — a, c, e
21. True — d
22. True — a, d, e
23. True — a, c
24. True — d, e
25. True — a
26. True — a, b, d
27. True — a, b
28. True — a, b, c, d, e
29. True — a, b, c, d
30. True — a, b

31. True — a, c
32. True — b, c, d
33. True — a, d, e
34. True — d, e
35. True — a, b, c, d, e
36. True — a, d
37. True — d, e
38. True — b, d, e
39. True — a, c, d, e
40. True — a, b
41. True — a, b, c, d, e
42. True — b, c, d
43. True — b, c, d
44. True — a, c
45. True — a, b, c, d
46. True — d
47. True — c, d
48. True — c, e
49. True — a, b, c, d
50. True — a, b, c, d, e
51. True — b, d
52. True — a, c, e
53. True — b, e
54. True — b, c, d, e
55. True — a, b, e
56. True — b, c, d
57. True — b, c, e
58. True — b, d
59. True — a, b, c
60. True — c, d, e